THE ART OF BECOMING ISN'T ABOUT PERFECTION - IT'S ABOUT INTENTIONAL GROWTH, SELF-LOVE, AND STEPPING INTO THE HIGHEST VERSION OF YOURSELF. THIS JOURNAL IS YOUR DAILY GUIDE TO TRANSFORMATION, HELPING YOU BUILD CONFIDENCE, RADIATE FEMININE ENERGY, AND CREATE A LIFESTYLE THAT ALIGNS WITH YOUR DREAMS AND GOALS.

INSIDE, YOU WILL FIND 180 DAILY AFFIRMATIONS DESIGNED TO REWIRE YOUR MINDSET, BOOST YOUR SELF-WORTH, AND KEEP YOU MOTIVATED. BUT THIS ISN'T JUST ABOUT READING WORDS - IT'S ABOUT EMBODYING THEM. EACH DAY, YOU'LL HAVE SPACE TO REFLECT, SET INTENTIONS, AND TRACK YOUR PROGRESS.

WHETHER YOU ARE STARTING FRESH, LEVELING UP, OR STEPPING DEEPER INTO YOUR GLOW-UP JOURNEY, THIS JOURNAL WILL BE YOUR DAILY DOSE OF INSPIRATION AND ACCOUNTABILITY. YOUR DREAM LIFE IS ALREADY YOURS - YOU JUST HAVE TO ALIGN WITH IT.

The Art of Becoming

DAY 1

DAILY CHECK IN: ✓

- WOKE UP EARLY ☐
- WENT TO THE GYM ☐
- MORNING ROUTINE ☐
- NIGHT ROUTINE ☐
- ATE HEALTHY WHOLE FOODS ☐
- READ AT LEAST 10 PAGES OF ANY BOOK ☐

7 DAYS MINDSET CHALLENGE
DAY 1

WRITE DOWN 3 LIMITING BELIEFS
AND REWRITE THEM
AS POSITIVE AFFIRMATIONS

REFLECTIION:

_____
_____
_____
_____
_____
_____
_____
_____

TODAY'S AFFIRMATION

I TRUST IN MY ABILITY TO CREATE THE LIFE I DESIRE. EVERY DECISION I MAKE AND EVERY STEP I TAKE BRINGS ME CLOSER TO MY DREAM LIFE.

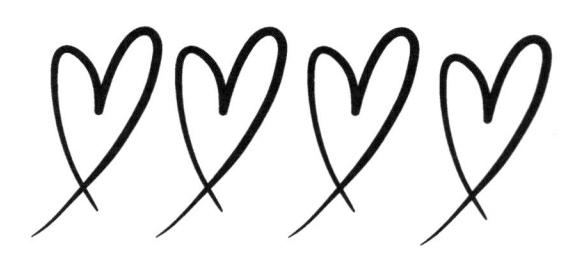

♡ ♡ ♡ ♡

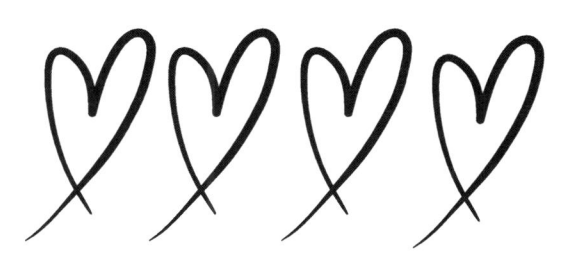

The Art of Becoming

DAY 2

DAILY CHECK IN: ✓

- WOKE UP EARLY
- WENT TO THE GYM
- MORNING ROUTINE
- NIGHT ROUTINE
- ATE HEALTHY WHOLE FOODS
- READ AT LEAST 10 PAGES OF ANY BOOK

7 DAYS MINDSET CHALLENGE
DAY 2

PRACTICE GRATITUDE
BY
LISTING 5 THINGS
YOU
ARE GRSTEFUL FOR

REFLECTIION:

_____
_____
_____
_____
_____
_____
_____
_____

TODAY'S AFFIRMATION

EVERY DAY, I BECOME
A
BETTER VERSION
OF MYSELF

♡ ♡ ♡ ♡

DAY 3

The Art of Becoming

DAILY CHECK IN: ✓

- WOKE UP EARLY ☐
- WENT TO THE GYM ☐
- MORNING ROUTINE ☐
- NIGHT ROUTINE ☐
- ATE HEALTHY WHOLE FOODS ☐
- READ AT LEAST 10 PAGES OF ANY BOOK ☐

7 DAYS MINDSET CHALLENGE
DAY 3

MEDITATE FOR 5-10 MINUTES
TO CLEAR YOUR MIND
OR
FAST FOR THE WHOLE DAY
IF YOU ARE ABLE TO,
BREAK YOUR FAST IN THE
EVENING, AROUND 7PM

REFLECTIION: _____

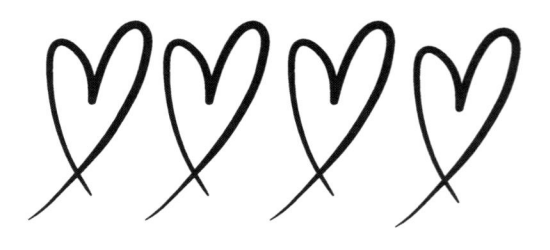

_____
_____
_____
_____
_____
_____
_____
_____
_____

TODAY'S AFFIRMATION

I AM
WORTHY
OF
LOVE, SUCCESS,
AND
HAPPINESS

DAY 4

The Art of Becoming

DAILY CHECK IN: ✓

- WOKE UP EARLY
- WENT TO THE GYM
- MORNING ROUTINE
- NIGHT ROUTINE
- ATE HEALTHY WHOLE FOODS
- READ AT LEAST 10 PAGES OF ANY BOOK

7 DAYS MINDSET CHALLENGE
DAY 4

DO SOMETHING
OUTSIDE
YOUR COMFORT
ZONE

REFLECTIION:

_____
_____
_____
_____
_____
_____
_____
_____
_____

TODAY'S AFFIRMATION

I
RADIATE
CONFIDENCE
AND
SELF-ASSURANCE

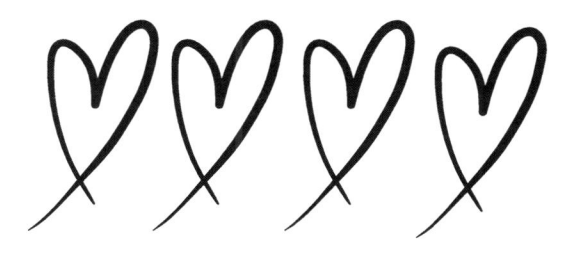

DAY 5

The Art of Becoming

DAILY CHECK IN: ✓

- WOKE UP EARLY
- WENT TO THE GYM
- MORNING ROUTINE
- NIGHT ROUTINE
- ATE HEALTHY WHOLE FOODS
- READ AT LEAST 10 PAGES OF ANY BOOK

7 DAYS MINDSET CHALLENGE
DAY 5

JOURNAL ABOUT
YOUR FUTURE SELF
AND
HER HABITS

REFLECTIION:

_____
_____
_____
_____
_____
_____
_____
_____

TODAY'S AFFIRMATION

MY
FEMININE ENERGY
IS
POWERFUL
AND
MAGNETIC

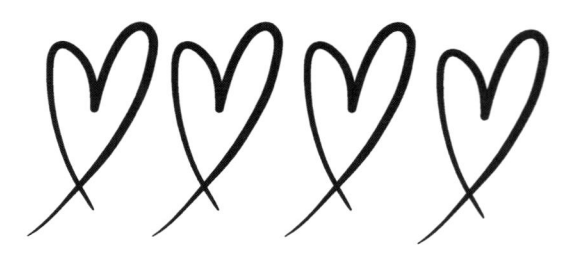

DAY 6

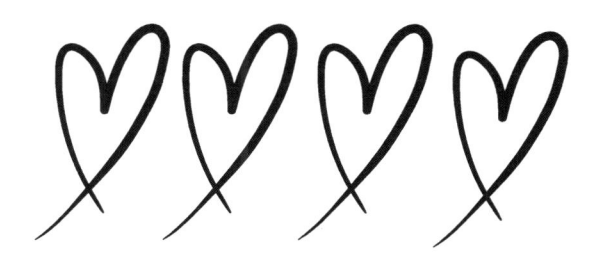

The Art of Becoming

DAILY CHECK IN: ✓

- WOKE UP EARLY
- WENT TO THE GYM
- MORNING ROUTINE
- NIGHT ROUTINE
- ATE HEALTHY WHOLE FOODS
- READ AT LEAST 10 PAGES OF ANY BOOK

7 DAYS MINDSET CHALLENGE
DAY 6

AVOID COMPLAINING FOR THE WHOLE DAY

REFLECTIION:

_____
_____
_____
_____
_____
_____
_____
_____
_____
_____

TODAY'S AFFIRMATION

I CHOOSE TO SEE CHALLENGES AS OPPORTUNITIES FOR GROWTH.

DAY 7

The Art of Becoming

DAILY CHECK IN: ✓

- WOKE UP EARLY ☐
- WENT TO THE GYM ☐
- MORNING ROUTINE ☐
- NIGHT ROUTINE ☐
- ATE HEALTHY WHOLE FOODS ☐
- READ AT LEAST 10 PAGES OF ANY BOOK ☐

7 DAYS MINDSET CHALLENGE
DAY 7

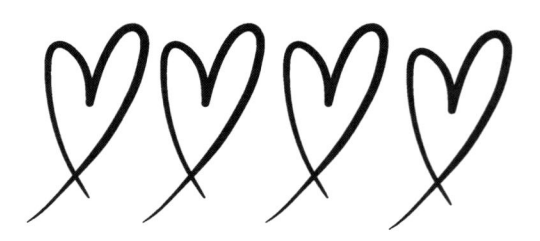

SPERAK ONLY POSITIVE WORDS ABOUT YOURSELF. HYPE UP YOUR OWN SELF.

REFLECTIION:

_____
_____
_____
_____
_____
_____
_____
_____
_____

TODAY'S AFFIRMATION

I AM DEEPLY LOVED AND SUPPORTED IN ALL AREAS OF MY LIFE.

DAY 8

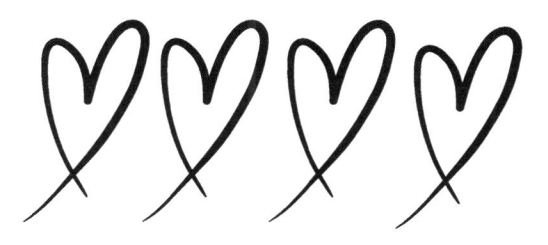

The Art of Becoming

DAILY CHECK IN: ✓

- WOKE UP EARLY
- WENT TO THE GYM
- MORNING ROUTINE
- NIGHT ROUTINE
- ATE HEALTHY WHOLE FOODS
- READ AT LEAST 10 PAGES OF ANY BOOK

TODAY'S AFFIRMATION

I PRIORITIZE MY WELL-BEING AND SELF-CARE

7 DAYS OF DECLUTTER
DAY 1

DECLUTTER YOUR CLOSET AND/OR KITCHEN. REMOVE ANYTHING THAT'S NO LONGER NEEDED. DONATE OR SELL ITEMS IN GOOD CONDITION

REFLECTIION:

_____
_____
_____
_____
_____
_____
_____
_____
_____

The Art of Becoming

DAY 9

DAILY CHECK IN ✓

- WOKE UP EARLY ☐
- WENT TO THE GYM ☐
- MORNING ROUTINE ☐
- NIGHT ROUTINE ☐
- ATE HEALTHY WHOLE FOODS ☐
- READ AT LEAST 10 PAGES OF ANY BOOK ☐

7 DAYS OF DECLUTTER
DAY2

DIGITAL DETOX:
DECLUTTER YOUR PHONE AND LAPTOP
DELETE UNUSED APPS, OLD PHOTOS AND UNNECESSARY DOWNLOADS.
UNSUBSCRIBE FROM SPAM MAILS AND ORGANIZE FILES INTO PROPER FOLDERS

REFLECTIION: _____
_____
_____
_____
_____
_____
_____
_____
_____

TODAY'S AFFIRMATION

I ATTRRACT ABUNDANCE IN ALL FORMS EFFORTLESSLY

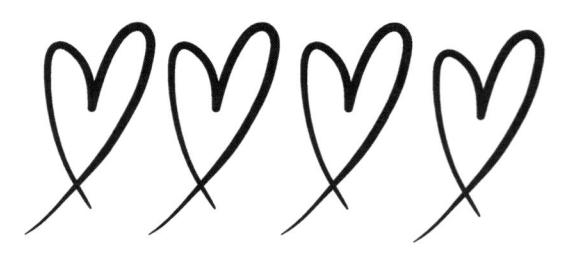

♡ ♡ ♡ ♡

The Art of Becoming

DAY 10

DAILY CHECK IN: ✓

- WOKE UP EARLY
- WENT TO THE GYM
- MORNING ROUTINE
- NIGHT ROUTINE
- ATE HEALTHY WHOLE FOODS
- READ AT LEAST 10 PAGES OF ANY BOOK

7 DAYS OF DECLUTTER
DAY 3

WARDROBE RESET:
REMOVE CLOTHES THAT DON'T FIT, DON'T MATCH YOUR STYLE ANYMORE.
CREATE 3 PILES: KEEP, DONATE, SELL
CREATE SPACE FOR NEW CLOTHES THAT ALIGN WITH YOUR NEW SELF

REFLECTIION:

_____
_____
_____
_____
_____
_____
_____
_____
_____

TODAY'S AFFIRMATION

I
AM
STEPPING INTO
MY POWER
WITH
CONFIDENCE AND
GRACE

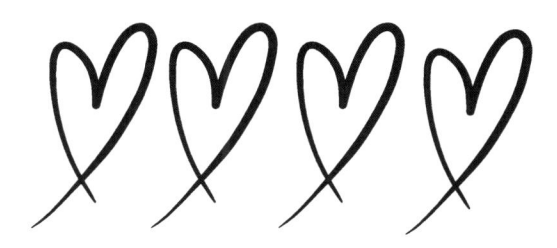

DAY 11

The Art of Becoming

DAILY CHECK IN: ✓

- WOKE UP EARLY ☐
- WENT TO THE GYM ☐
- MORNING ROUTINE ☐
- NIGHT ROUTINE ☐
- ATE HEALTHY WHOLE FOODS ☐
- READ AT LEAST 10 PAGES OF ANY BOOK ☐

7 DAYS OF DECLUTTER
DAY 4

MENTAL DECLUTTER:
IDENTIFY WHAT'S SERVING YOU VS. WHAT'S DRAINING YOU.
SET CLEAR INTENTIONS FOR A FRESH START.
TRY A SHORT MEDITATION OR DEEP BREATHING TO RESET.

REFLECTIION:

_____
_____
_____
_____
_____
_____
_____
_____

TODAY'S AFFIRMATION

I AM STEPPING INTO MY POWER, KNOWING I AM CAPABLE OF ACHIEVING ANYTHING

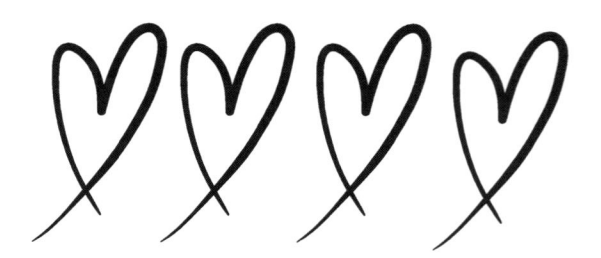

DAY 12

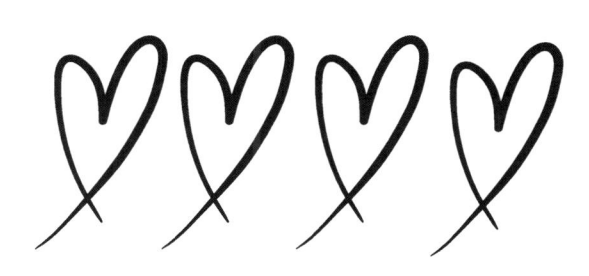

The Art of Becoming

DAILY CHECK IN: ✓

- WOKE UP EARLY
- WENT TO THE GYM
- MORNING ROUTINE
- NIGHT ROUTINE
- ATE HEALTHY WHOLE FOODS
- READ AT LEAST 10 PAGES OF ANY BOOK

7 DAYS OF DECLUTTER
DAY 5

SOCIAL CLEANSE: SET BOUNDARIES
UNFOLLOW OR MUTE TOXIC SOCIAL MEDIA ACCOUNTS.
SET BOUNDARIES WITH PEOPLE WHO OVERSTEP
SPEND INTENTIONAL TIME WITH UPLIFTING PEOPLE.

REFLECTIION:

_____
_____
_____
_____
_____
_____
_____
_____
_____

TODAY'S AFFIRMATION

CONFIDENCE
IS A SKILL
I
BUILD DAILY BY
SHOWING UP AS MY
BEST SELF

♡ ♡ ♡ ♡

The Art of Becoming

DAY 13

DAILY CHECK IN: ✓

- WOKE UP EARLY
- WENT TO THE GYM
- MORNING ROUTINE
- NIGHT ROUTINE
- ATE HEALTHY WHOLE FOODS
- READ AT LEAST 10 PAGES OF ANY BOOK

7 DAYS OF DECLUTTER
DAY 6

FINANCIAL DECLUTTER:
ORGANIZE MONEY AND EXPENSES
REVIEW SUBSCRIPTIONS AND CANCEL ANYTHING UNNECESSARY.
ORGANIZE YOUR WALLET (REMOVE OLD RECEIPTS, EXPIRED CARDS)

REFLECTIION:

_____
_____
_____
_____
_____
_____
_____
_____

TODAY'S AFFIRMATION

I RELEASE ALL FEAR AND SELF-DOUBT BECAUSE I TRUST MY OWN GROWTH.

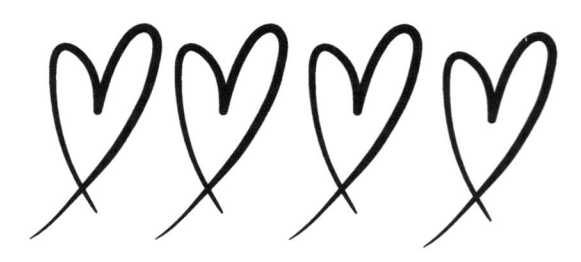

DAY 14

The Art of Becoming

DAILY CHECK IN: ✓

- WOKE UP EARLY
- WENT TO THE GYM
- MORNING ROUTINE
- NIGHT ROUTINE
- ATE HEALTHY WHOLE FOODS
- READ AT LEAST 10 PAGES OF ANY BOOK

7 DAYS OF DECLUTTER
DAY 7

ENERGY DETOX:
REFRESH YOUR SPACE
BURN
SAGE,
OR LIGHT A CANDLE
FOR
FRESH ENERGY

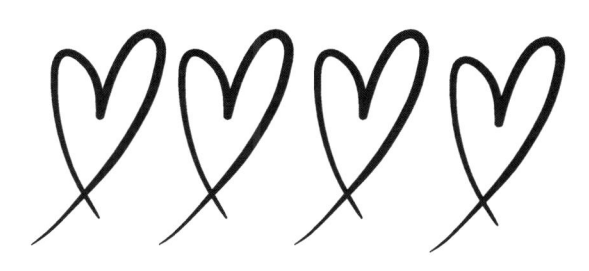

REFLECTIION:
_____
_____
_____
_____
_____
_____
_____
_____
_____

TODAY'S AFFIRMATION

I ALLOW MYSELF TO TAKE UP SPACE, KNOWING I AM WORTHY OF BEING SEEN AND HEARD

The Art of Becoming

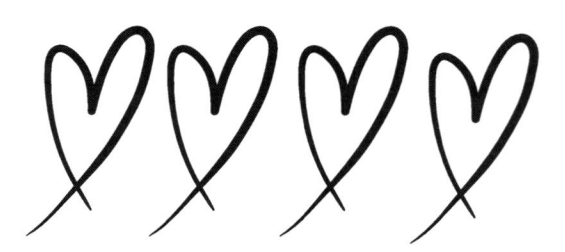

DAY 15

DAILY CHECK IN: ✓

- WOKE UP EARLY ☐
- WENT TO THE GYM ☐
- MORNING ROUTINE ☐
- NIGHT ROUTINE ☐
- ATE HEALTHY WHOLE FOODS ☐
- READ AT LEAST 10 PAGES OF ANY BOOK ☐

7 DAYS CHALLENGE OF CURATING MY SIGNATURE AESTHETIC

DAY 1

DEFINE YOUR AESTHETIC
CREATE A PINTEREST MOOD BOARD WITH OUTFIT INSPIRATIONS.
FIND STYLE MUSES WHO INSPIRE YOU.

REFLECTIION:
_____
_____
_____
_____
_____
_____
_____
_____

TODAY'S AFFIRMATION

I NO LONGER SEEK VALIDATION FROM OTHERS
- I VALIDATE MYSELF.

The Art of Becoming

DAY 16

DAILY CHECK IN: ✓

- WOKE UP EARLY
- WENT TO THE GYM
- MORNING ROUTINE
- NIGHT ROUTINE
- ATE HEALTHY WHOLE FOODS
- READ AT LEAST 10 PAGES OF ANY BOOK

7 DAYS CHALLENGE OF CURATING MY SIGNATURE AESTHETIC
DAY 2

DECLUTTER AND EDIT YOUR CLOSET
REMOVE ANYTHING THAT DOESNT FIT, FLATTER, OR ALIGN WITH YOUR NEW AESTHETIC

REFLECTIION: _____
_____
_____
_____
_____
_____
_____
_____
_____
_____

TODAY'S AFFIRMATION

I AM NO LONGER AFRAID OF FAILURE;
I SEE IT AS A STEPPING STONE TO SUCCESS

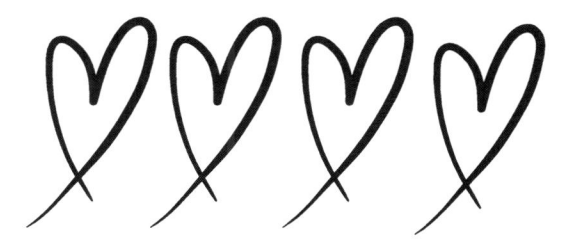

♡ ♡ ♡ ♡

The Art of Becoming

DAY 17

DAILY CHECK IN: ✓

- WOKE UP EARLY ☐
- WENT TO THE GYM ☐
- MORNING ROUTINE ☐
- NIGHT ROUTINE ☐
- ATE HEALTHY WHOLE FOODS ☐
- READ AT LEAST 10 PAGES OF ANY BOOK ☐

7 DAYS CHALLENGE OF CURATING MY SIGNATURE AESTHETIC

DAY 3

FIND YOUR SIGNATURE COLORS AND SILHOUETTES
IDENTIFY COLORS THAT COMPLEMENT YOUR SKIN TONE AND BRING OUT YOUR FEATURES.

REFLECTIION:
_____
_____
_____
_____
_____
_____
_____
_____
_____

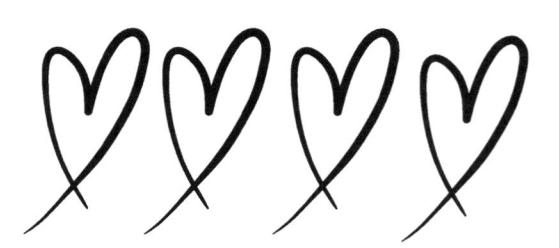

TODAY'S AFFIRMATION

EVERY SMALL STEP I TAKE LEADS ME CLOSER TO MY HIGHEST SELF.

♡ ♡ ♡ ♡

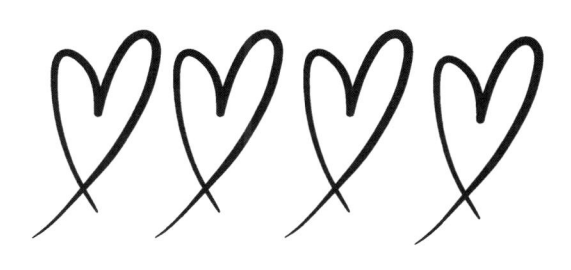

The Art of Becoming

DAY 18

DAILY CHECK IN: ✓

- WOKE UP EARLY
- WENT TO THE GYM
- MORNING ROUTINE
- NIGHT ROUTINE
- ATE HEALTHY WHOLE FOODS
- READ AT LEAST 10 PAGES OF ANY BOOK

7 DAYS CHALLENGE OF CURATING MY SIGNATURE AESTHETIC

DAY 4

UPGRADE YOUR WARDROBE ESSENTIALS
INVEST IN QUALITY OVER QUANTITY - FOCUS ON TIMELESS, VERSATILE STAPLES
LOOK FOR BRANDS THAT ALIGN WITH YOUR AESTHETIC.

REFLECTIION:
_____
_____
_____
_____
_____
_____
_____
_____
_____

TODAY'S AFFIRMATION

I AM DONE SHRINKING MYSELF TO FIT IN - I AM HERE TO STAND OUT

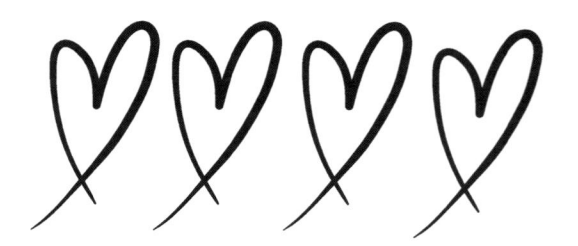

The Art of Becoming

DAY 19

DAILY CHECK IN: ✓

- WOKE UP EARLY ☐
- WENT TO THE GYM ☐
- MORNING ROUTINE ☐
- NIGHT ROUTINE ☐
- ATE HEALTHY WHOLE FOODS ☐
- READ AT LEAST 10 PAGES OF ANY BOOK ☐

7 DAYS CHALLENGE OF CURATING MY SIGNATURE AESTHETIC
DAY5

ELEVATE YOUR BEAUTY AND GROOMING ROUTINE
FIND A SIGNATURE HAIRSTYLE AND MAKEUP LOOK THAT BEST SUITS YOU.
PRIORITIZE SKINCARE AND SELF-CARE FOR THAT EFFORTLESS GLOW.

REFLECTIION: _____
_____
_____
_____
_____
_____
_____
_____
_____

TODAY'S AFFIRMATION

I
HONOR MY UNIQUE JOURNEY
AND TRUST MY OWN TIMING

DAY 20

The Art of Becoming

7 DAYS CHALLENGE OF CURATING MY OWN SIGNATURE AESTHETIC

DAY 6

DAILY CHECK IN: ✓

- WOKE UP EARLY
- WENT TO THE GYM
- MORNING ROUTINE
- NIGHT ROUTINE
- ATE HEALTHY WHOLE FOODS
- READ AT LEAST 10 PAGES OF ANY BOOK

CURATE YOUR ACCESSORIES AND PERSONAL TOUCH
CHOOSE JEWELRY, HANDBAGS, AND SHOES THAT ALIGN WITH YOUR AESTHETIC
KEEP IT MINIMAL YET IMPACTFUL - LESS BUT BETTER

REFLECTIION:
_____
_____
_____
_____
_____
_____
_____
_____
_____

TODAY'S AFFIRMATION

I WELCOME NEW OPPORTUNITIES, KNOWING THEY ARE MEANT FOR ME.

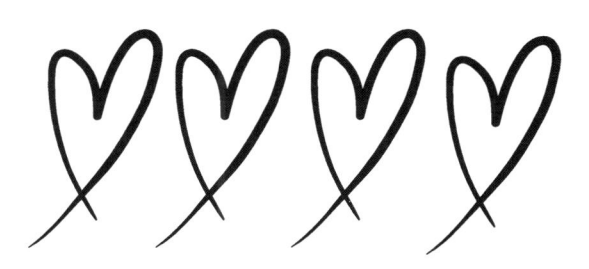

The Art of Becoming

DAY 21

DAILY CHECK IN: ✓

- WOKE UP EARLY
- WENT TO THE GYM
- MORNING ROUTINE
- NIGHT ROUTINE
- ATE HEALTHY WHOLE FOODS
- READ AT LEAST 10 PAGES OF ANY BOOK

7 DAYS CHALLENGE OF CURATING MY SIGNATURE AESTHETIC

DAY 7

EMBODY YOUR AESTHETIC DAILY
PUT TOGETHER A FULL OUTFIT THAT REPRESENTS YOUR CURATED LOOK
WALK WITH CONFIDENCE
OWN YOUR STYLE AND LET IT EVOLVE NATURALLY

REFLECTIION:

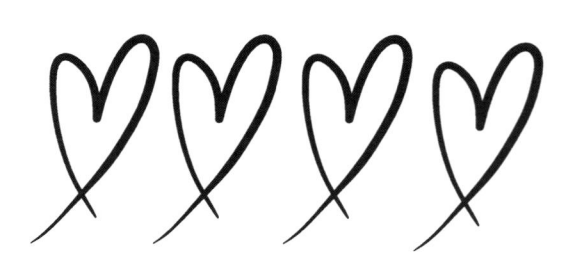

_____
_____
_____
_____
_____
_____
_____
_____
_____

TODAY'S AFFIRMATION

I AM FEARLESS IN THE PURSUIT OF WHAT SETS MY SOUL ON FIRE.

The Art of Becoming

DAY 22

DAILY CHECK IN: ✓

- WOKE UP EARLY
- WENT TO THE GYM
- MORNING ROUTINE
- NIGHT ROUTINE
- ATE HEALTHY WHOLE FOODS
- READ AT LEAST 10 PAGES OF ANY BOOK

REFLECTIION:

_____
_____
_____
_____
_____
_____
_____
_____
_____

TODAY'S AFFIRMATION

I AM STRONGER THAN MY FEARS AND DOUBTS.

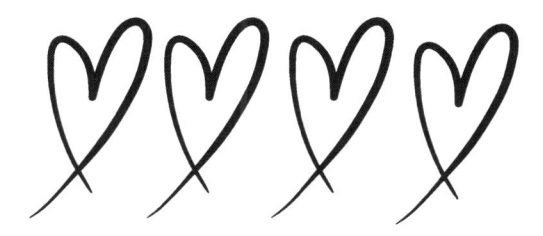

♡ ♡ ♡ ♡

The Art of Becoming

DAY 23

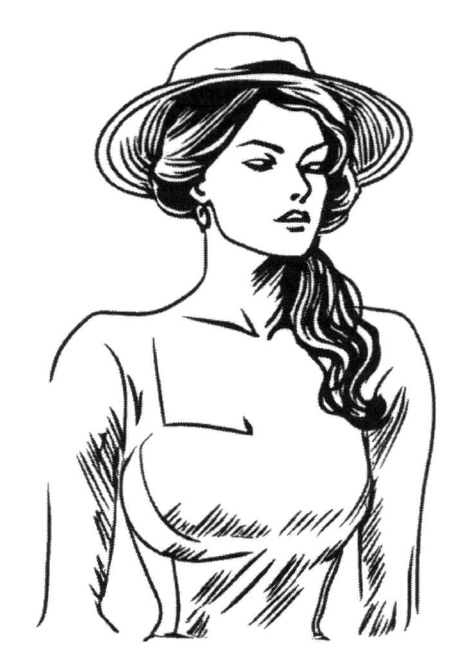

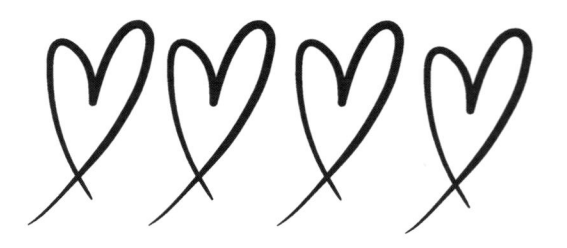

DAILY CHECK IN: ✓

- WOKE UP EARLY
- WENT TO THE GYM
- MORNING ROUTINE
- NIGHT ROUTINE
- ATE HEALTHY WHOLE FOODS
- READ AT LEAST 10 PAGES OF ANY BOOK

REFLECTIION:
_____
_____
_____
_____
_____
_____
_____
_____
_____

TODAY'S AFFIRMATION

I BELIEVE IN MYSELF MORE THAN EVER NOW

♡ ♡ ♡ ♡

The Art of Becoming

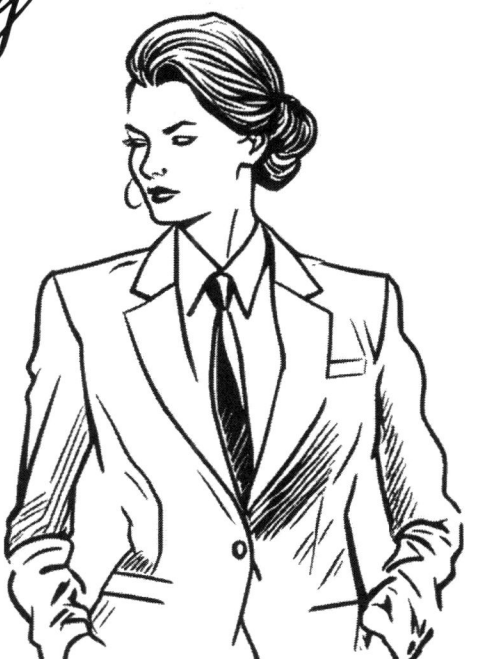

DAY 24

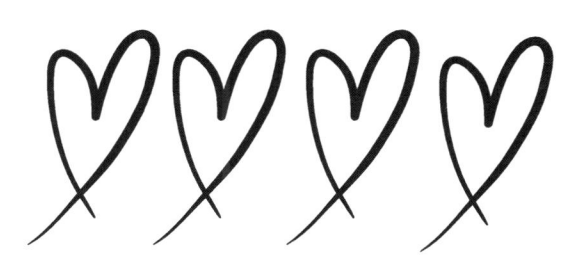

DAILY CHECK IN: ✓

- WOKE UP EARLY
- WENT TO THE GYM
- MORNING ROUTINE
- NIGHT ROUTINE
- ATE HEALTHY WHOLE FOODS
- READ AT LEAST 10 PAGES OF ANY BOOK

REFLECTIION:

_____
_____
_____
_____
_____
_____
_____
_____
_____

TODAY'S AFFIRMATION

I KNOW MY WORTH AND I WILL NEVER AGAIN SETTLE FOR LESS THAN I DESERVE

The Art of Becoming

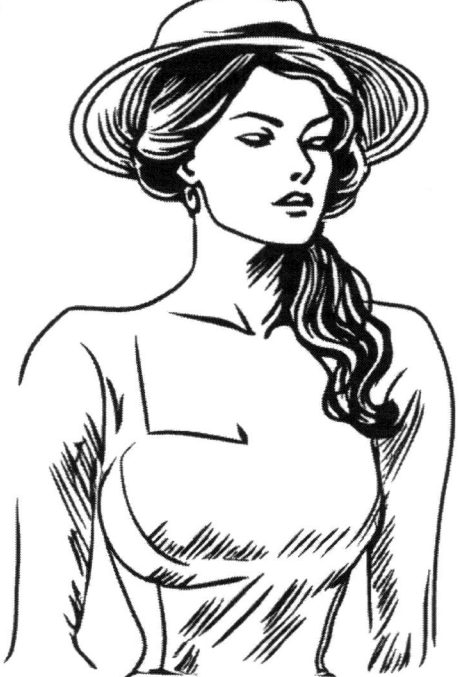

DAY 25

DAILY CHECK IN: ✓

- WOKE UP EARLY ☐
- WENT TO THE GYM ☐
- MORNING ROUTINE ☐
- NIGHT ROUTINE ☐
- ATE HEALTHY WHOLE FOODS ☐
- READ AT LEAST 10 PAGES OF ANY BOOK ☐

REFLECTIION:

_____
_____
_____
_____
_____
_____
_____
_____
_____

TODAY'S AFFIRMATION

I DESERVE SUCCESS, HAPPINESS, AND ABUNDANCE

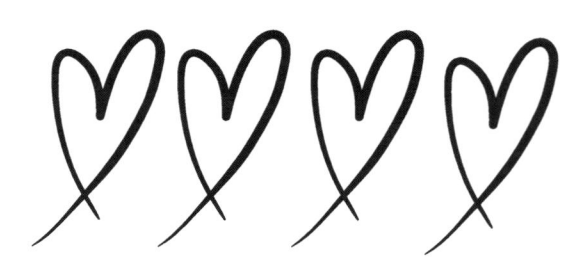

♡ ♡ ♡ ♡

The Art of Becoming

DAY 26

DAILY CHECK IN: ✓

- WOKE UP EARLY
- WENT TO THE GYM
- MORNING ROUTINE
- NIGHT ROUTINE
- ATE HEALTHY WHOLE FOODS
- READ AT LEAST 10 PAGES OF ANY BOOK

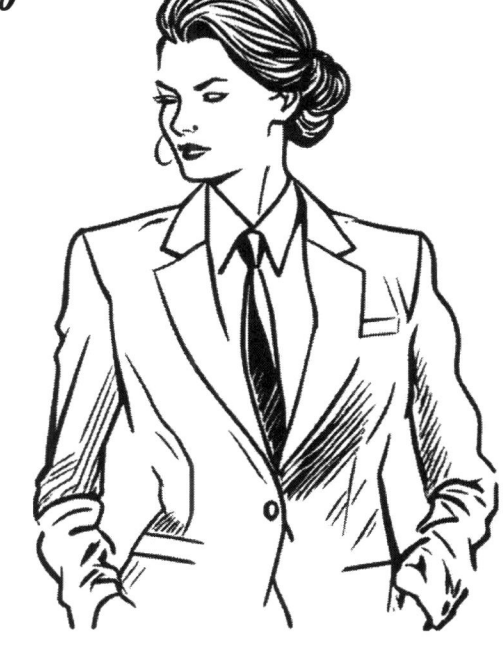

REFLECTIION:
_____
_____
_____
_____
_____
_____
_____
_____
_____

TODAY'S AFFIRMATION

I AM BOLD ENOUGH TO GO AFTER WHAT I WANT

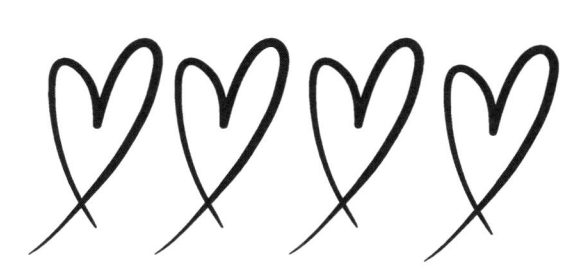

The Art of Becoming

DAY 27

DAILY CHECK IN: ✓

- WOKE UP EARLY
- WENT TO THE GYM
- MORNING ROUTINE
- NIGHT ROUTINE
- ATE HEALTHY WHOLE FOODS
- READ AT LEAST 10 PAGES OF ANY BOOK

REFLECTIION:

_____
_____
_____
_____
_____
_____
_____
_____

TODAY'S AFFIRMATION

I RELEASE ALL LIMITATIONS AND STEP INTO MY FULL POTENTIAL

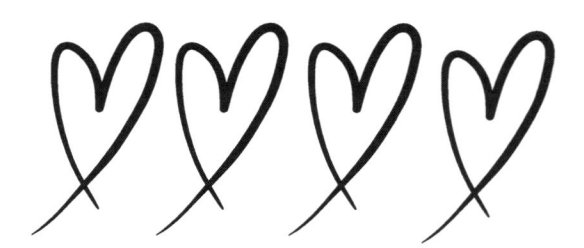

The Art of Becoming

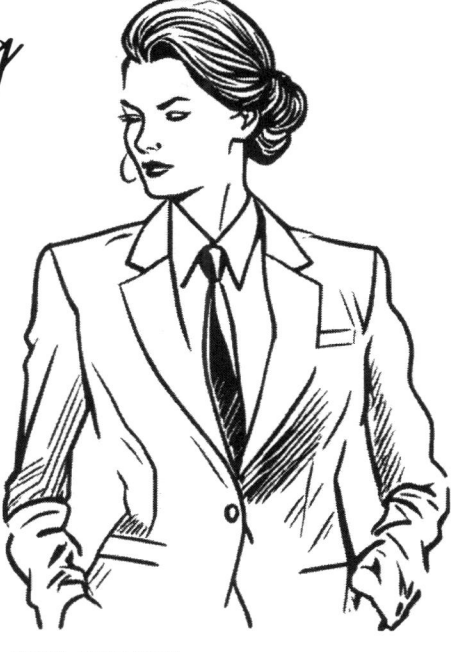

DAY 28

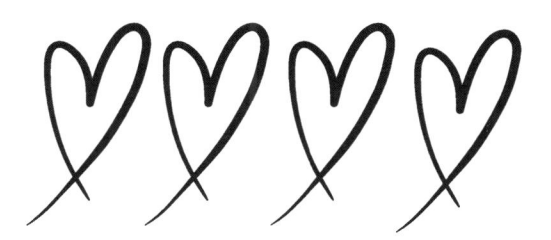

DAILY CHECK IN: ✓

- WOKE UP EARLY
- WENT TO THE GYM
- MORNING ROUTINE
- NIGHT ROUTINE
- ATE HEALTHY WHOLE FOODS
- READ AT LEAST 10 PAGES OF ANY BOOK

REFLECTIION:

_____
_____
_____
_____
_____
_____
_____
_____

TODAY'S AFFIRMATION

I AM PROUD OF THE WOMAN I AM BECOMING

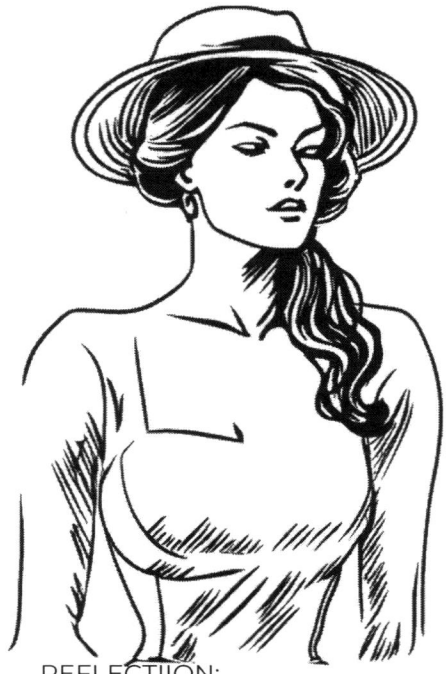

The Art of Becoming

DAY 29

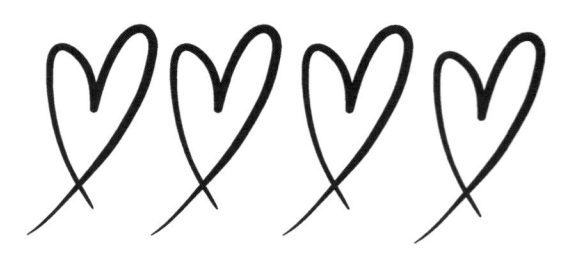

DAILY CHECK IN: ✓

- WOKE UP EARLY ☐
- WENT TO THE GYM ☐
- MORNING ROUTINE ☐
- NIGHT ROUTINE ☐
- ATE HEALTHY WHOLE FOODS ☐
- READ AT LEAST 10 PAGES OF ANY BOOK ☐

REFLECTIION:

_____
_____
_____
_____
_____
_____
_____
_____
_____

TODAY'S AFFIRMATION

I WAKE UP EVERYDAY WITH CONFIDENCE, CLARITY, AND PURPOSE

DAY 30

The Art of Becoming

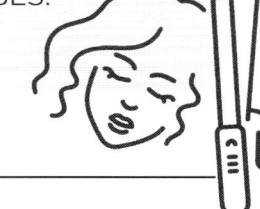

DAILY CHECK IN: ✓

- WOKE UP EARLY
- WENT TO THE GYM
- MORNING ROUTINE
- NIGHT ROUTINE
- ATE HEALTHY WHOLE FOODS
- READ AT LEAST 10 PAGES OF ANY BOOK

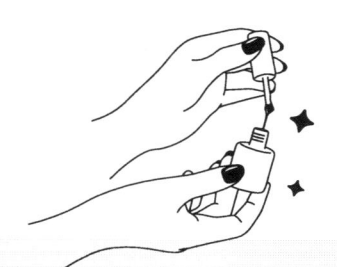

MAINTENANCE DAY
TIME
TO VISIT
THE BEAUTY PARLOR,
BABES!

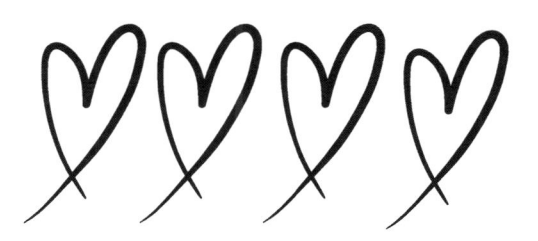

REFLECTIION:
_____
_____
_____
_____
_____
_____
_____
_____
_____

TODAY'S AFFIRMATION

I AM THAT GIRL -
RADIANT,
CONFIDENT, AND
UNSTOPPABLE

The Art of Becoming

DAY 31

DAILY CHECK IN: ✓

- WOKE UP EARLY
- WENT TO THE GYM
- MORNING ROUTINE
- NIGHT ROUTINE
- ATE HEALTHY WHOLE FOODS
- READ AT LEAST 10 PAGES OF ANY BOOK

REFLECTIION:

_____
_____
_____
_____
_____
_____
_____
_____
_____

TODAY'S AFFIRMATION

I AM WORTHY OF LOVE, RESPECT, AND ABUNDANCE

DAY 32

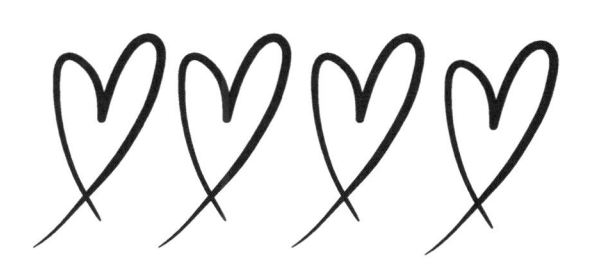

The Art of Becoming

DAILY CHECK IN: ✓

- WOKE UP EARLY
- WENT TO THE GYM
- MORNING ROUTINE
- NIGHT ROUTINE
- ATE HEALTHY WHOLE FOODS
- READ AT LEAST 10 PAGES OF ANY BOOK

REFLECTIION:

_____
_____
_____
_____
_____
_____
_____
_____
_____
_____

TODAY'S AFFIRMATION

I TAKE CARE OF MYSELF BEACAUSE I DESERVE TO FEEL MY BEST.

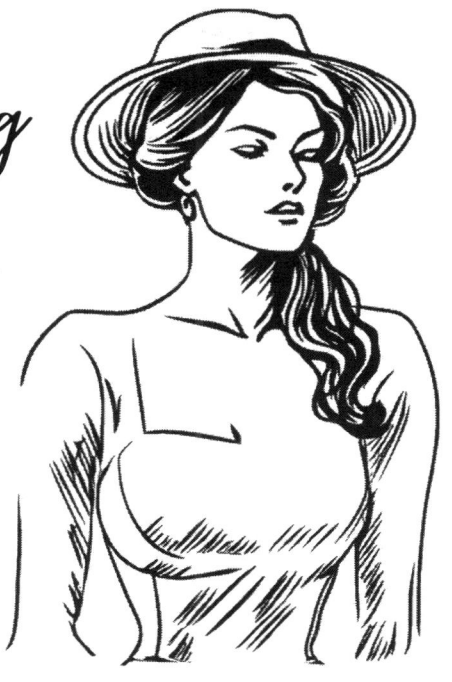

The Art of Becoming

DAY 33

DAILY CHECK IN: ✓

- WOKE UP EARLY
- WENT TO THE GYM
- MORNING ROUTINE
- NIGHT ROUTINE
- ATE HEALTHY WHOLE FOODS
- READ AT LEAST 10 PAGES OF ANY BOOK

REFLECTIION:

_____
_____
_____
_____
_____
_____
_____
_____
_____

TODAY'S AFFIRMATION

MY BODY IS MY TEMPLE, AND I NOURISH IT WITH LOVE AND CARE

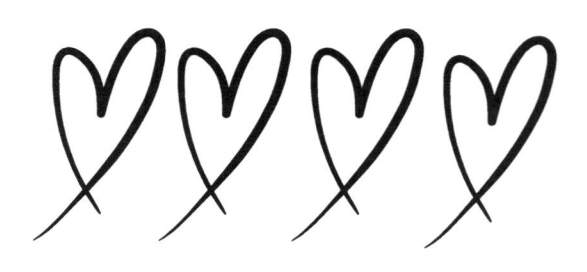

The Art of Becoming

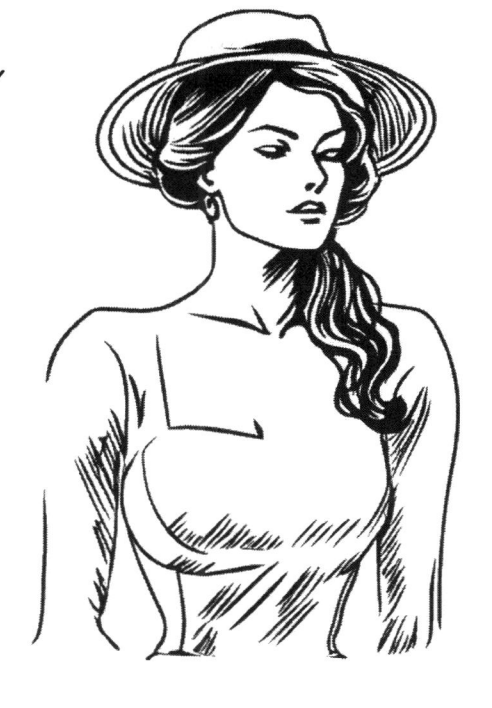

DAY 34

DAILY CHECK IN: ✓

- WOKE UP EARLY
- WENT TO THE GYM
- MORNING ROUTINE
- NIGHT ROUTINE
- ATE HEALTHY WHOLE FOODS
- READ AT LEAST 10 PAGES OF ANY BOOK

REFLECTIION:
_____
_____
_____
_____
_____
_____
_____
_____
_____

TODAY'S AFFIRMATION

I NOW SET HIGH STANDARDS BECAUSE I RESPECT MYSELF

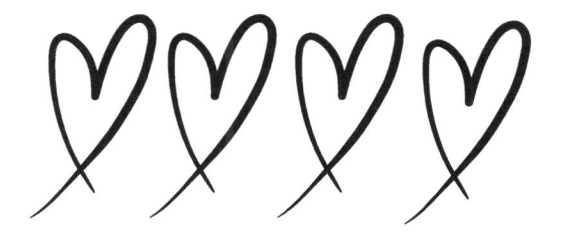

The Art of Becoming

DAY 35

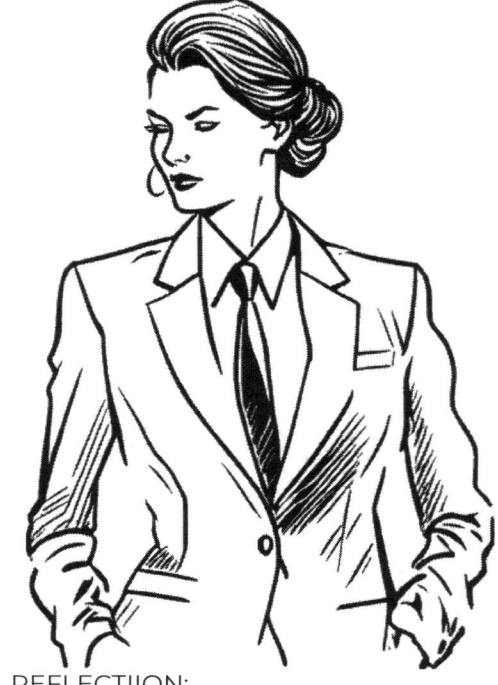

DAILY CHECK IN: ✓

- WOKE UP EARLY ☐
- WENT TO THE GYM ☐
- MORNING ROUTINE ☐
- NIGHT ROUTINE ☐
- ATE HEALTHY WHOLE FOODS ☐
- READ AT LEAST 10 PAGES OF ANY BOOK ☐

REFLECTIION:

_____
_____
_____
_____
_____
_____
_____
_____

TODAY'S AFFIRMATION

I AM KIND TO MYSELF, ALWAYS SPEAKING WITH LOVE AND ENCOURAGEMENT

The Art of Becoming

DAY 36

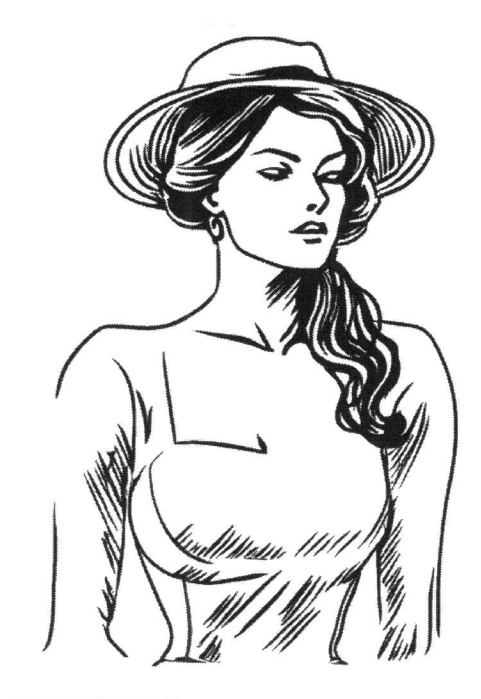

DAILY CHECK IN: ✓

- WOKE UP EARLY
- WENT TO THE GYM
- MORNING ROUTINE
- NIGHT ROUTINE
- ATE HEALTHY WHOLE FOODS
- READ AT LEAST 10 PAGES OF ANY BOOK

REFLECTIION:

TODAY'S AFFIRMATION

I HONOR MY BOUNDARIES AND PROTECT MY ENERGY,

The Art of Becoming

DAY 37

DAILY CHECK IN: ✓

- WOKE UP EARLY ☐
- WENT TO THE GYM ☐
- MORNING ROUTINE ☐
- NIGHT ROUTINE ☐
- ATE HEALTHY WHOLE FOODS ☐
- READ AT LEAST 10 PAGES OF ANY BOOK ☐

REFLECTIION:

_____
_____
_____
_____
_____
_____
_____
_____
_____

TODAY'S AFFIRMATION

I
LET GO OF
NEGATIVE SELF-TALK
AND
EMBRACE
SELF-LOVE

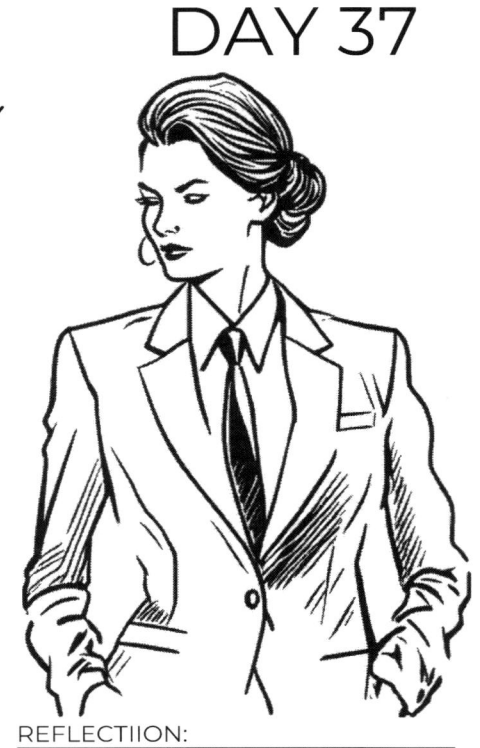

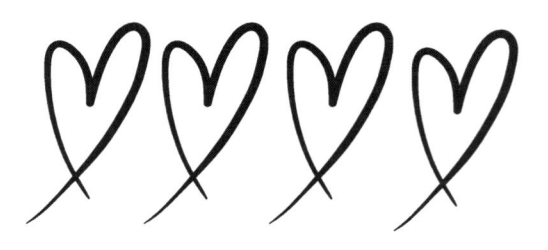

The Art of Becoming

DAY 38

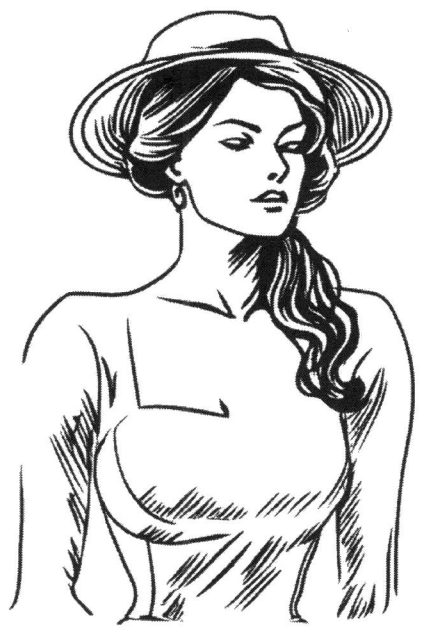

DAILY CHECK IN: ✓

- WOKE UP EARLY ☐
- WENT TO THE GYM ☐
- MORNING ROUTINE ☐
- NIGHT ROUTINE ☐
- ATE HEALTHY WHOLE FOODS ☐
- READ AT LEAST 10 PAGES OF ANY BOOK ☐

REFLECTIION:
_____
_____
_____
_____
_____
_____
_____
_____
_____

TODAY'S AFFIRMATION

I GIVE MYSELF PERMISSION TO REST WITHOUT GUILT

DAY 39

The Art of Becoming

DAILY CHECK IN: ✓

- WOKE UP EARLY ☐
- WENT TO THE GYM ☐
- MORNING ROUTINE ☐
- NIGHT ROUTINE ☐
- ATE HEALTHY WHOLE FOODS ☐
- READ AT LEAST 10 PAGES OF ANY BOOK ☐

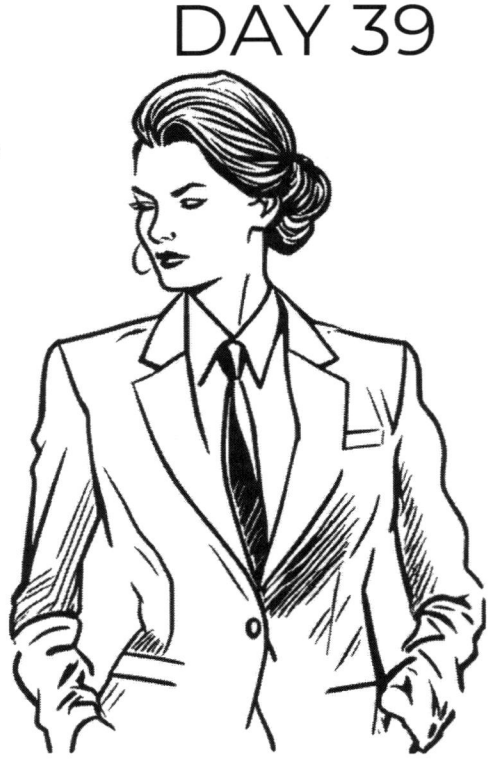

REFLECTIION:

_____
_____
_____
_____
_____
_____
_____
_____

TODAY'S AFFIRMATION

MY HAPPINESS IS MY RESPONSIBILITY, AND I CHOOSE JOY DAILY.

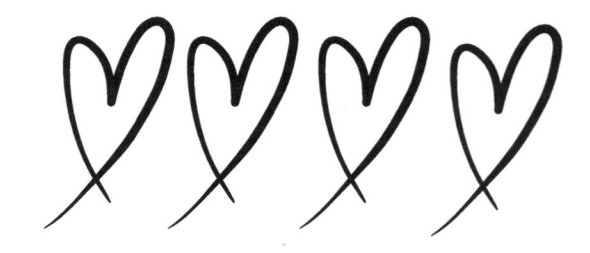

The Art of Becoming

DAY 40

DAILY CHECK IN: ✓

- WOKE UP EARLY
- WENT TO THE GYM
- MORNING ROUTINE
- NIGHT ROUTINE
- ATE HEALTHY WHOLE FOODS
- READ AT LEAST 10 PAGES OF ANY BOOK

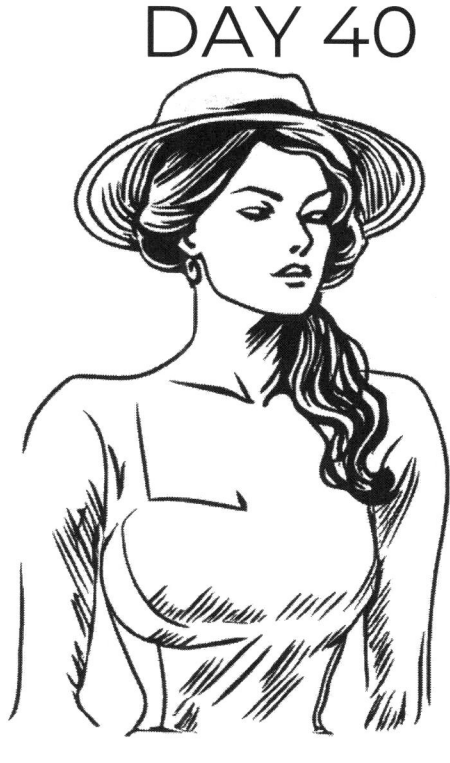

REFLECTIION:
_____
_____
_____
_____
_____
_____
_____
_____
_____

TODAY'S AFFIRMATION

I RADIATE BEAUTY, GRACE, AND CONFIDENCE FROM WITHIN

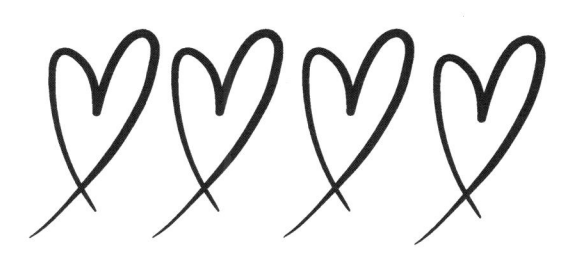

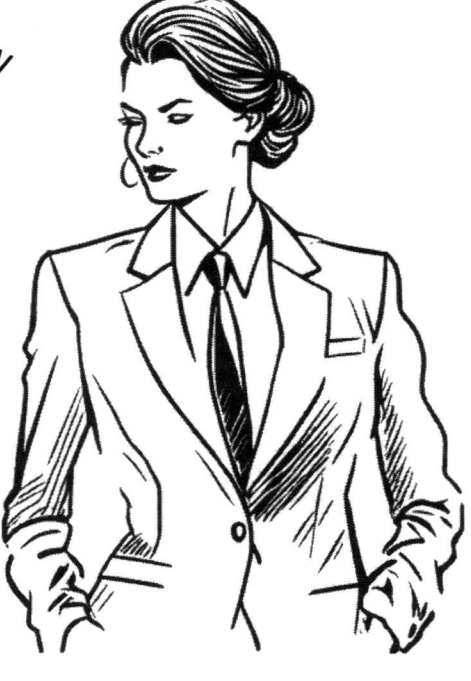

DAY 41

The Art of Becoming

DAILY CHECK IN: ✓

- WOKE UP EARLY
- WENT TO THE GYM
- MORNING ROUTINE
- NIGHT ROUTINE
- ATE HEALTHY WHOLE FOODS
- READ AT LEAST 10 PAGES OF ANY BOOK

REFLECTIION:

_____
_____
_____
_____
_____
_____
_____
_____

TODAY'S AFFIRMATION

I AM PATIENT WITH MYSELF AS I GROW AND EVOLVE

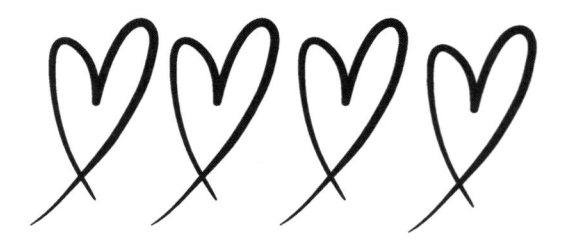

The Art of Becoming

DAY 42

DAILY CHECK IN: ✓

- WOKE UP EARLY
- WENT TO THE GYM
- MORNING ROUTINE
- NIGHT ROUTINE
- ATE HEALTHY WHOLE FOODS
- READ AT LEAST 10 PAGES OF ANY BOOK

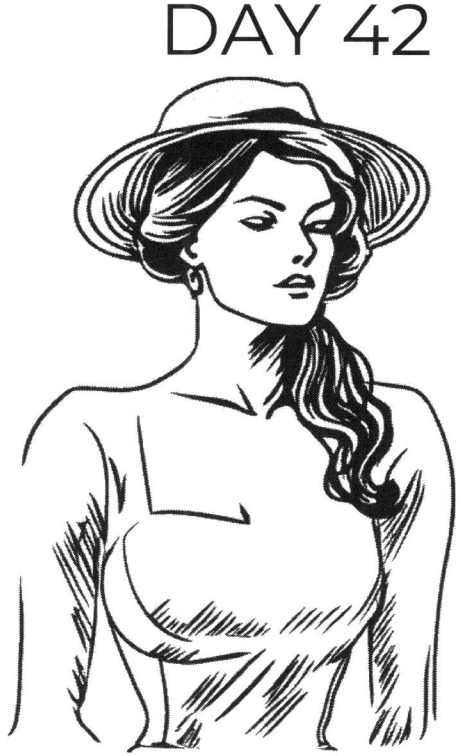

REFLECTIION:

_____
_____
_____
_____
_____
_____
_____
_____
_____

TODAY'S AFFIRMATION

I AM BECOMING AT PEACE WITH WHO I AM AND WHO I AM BECOMING

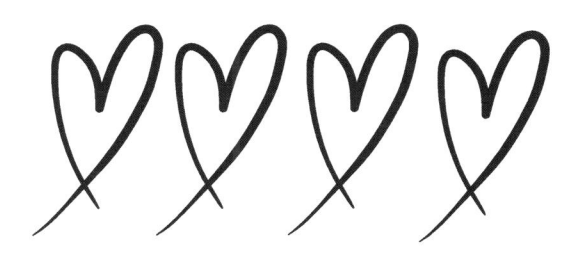

The Art of Becoming

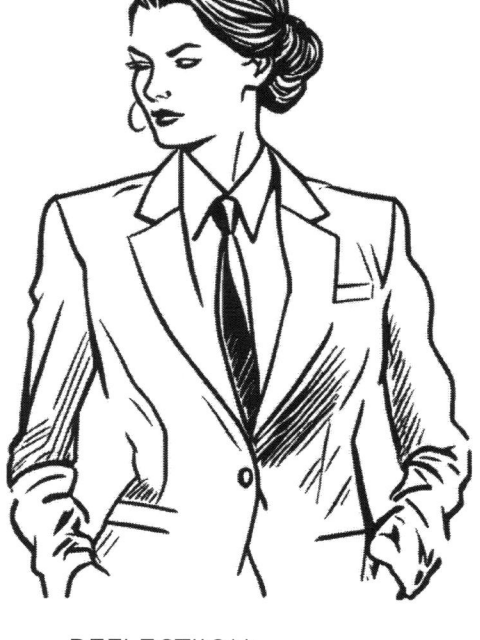

DAY 43

DAILY CHECK IN: ✓

- WOKE UP EARLY
- WENT TO THE GYM
- MORNING ROUTINE
- NIGHT ROUTINE
- ATE HEALTHY WHOLE FOODS
- READ AT LEAST 10 PAGES OF ANY BOOK

REFLECTIION:

_____
_____
_____
_____
_____
_____
_____
_____
_____

TODAY'S AFFIRMATION

I RELEASE PAST MISTAKES AND EMBRACE MY FRESH START

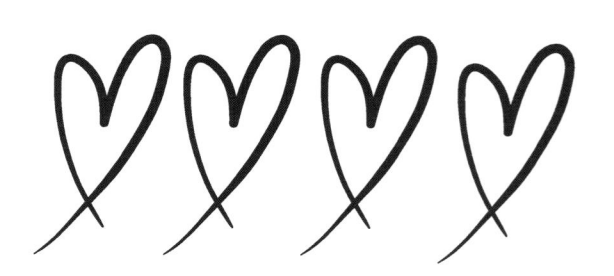

The Art of Becoming

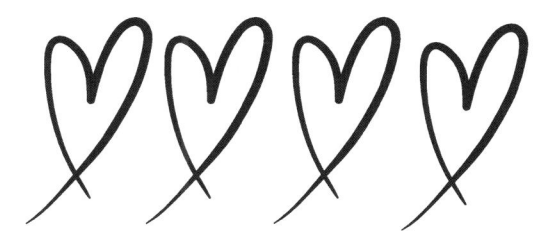

DAY 44

DAILY CHECK IN: ✓

- WOKE UP EARLY
- WENT TO THE GYM
- MORNING ROUTINE
- NIGHT ROUTINE
- ATE HEALTHY WHOLE FOODS
- READ AT LEAST 10 PAGES OF ANY BOOK

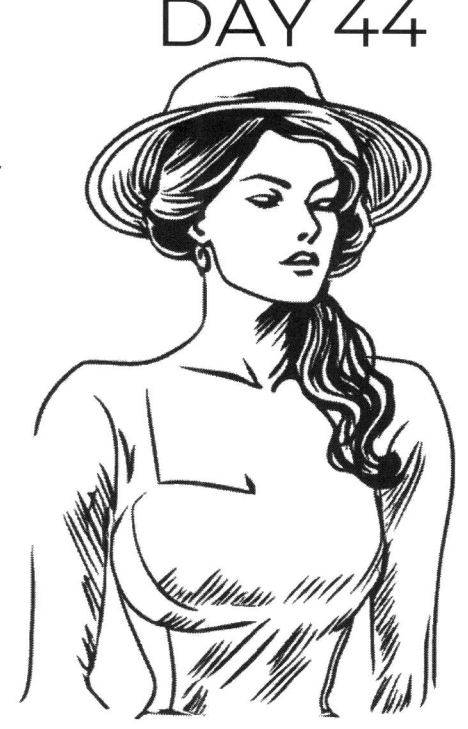

REFLECTIION:

_____
_____
_____
_____
_____
_____
_____
_____
_____

TODAY'S AFFIRMATION

I
AM PROUD
OF HOW FAR
I
HAVE COME

The Art of Becoming

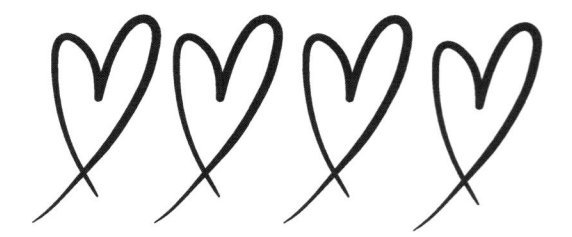

DAY 45

DAILY CHECK IN: ✓

- WOKE UP EARLY
- WENT TO THE GYM
- MORNING ROUTINE
- NIGHT ROUTINE
- ATE HEALTHY WHOLE FOODS
- READ AT LEAST 10 PAGES OF ANY BOOK

REFLECTIION:

_____
_____
_____
_____
_____
_____
_____
_____
_____

TODAY'S AFFIRMATION

I TREAT MYSELF WITH THE SAME KINDNESS I GIVE TO OTHERS

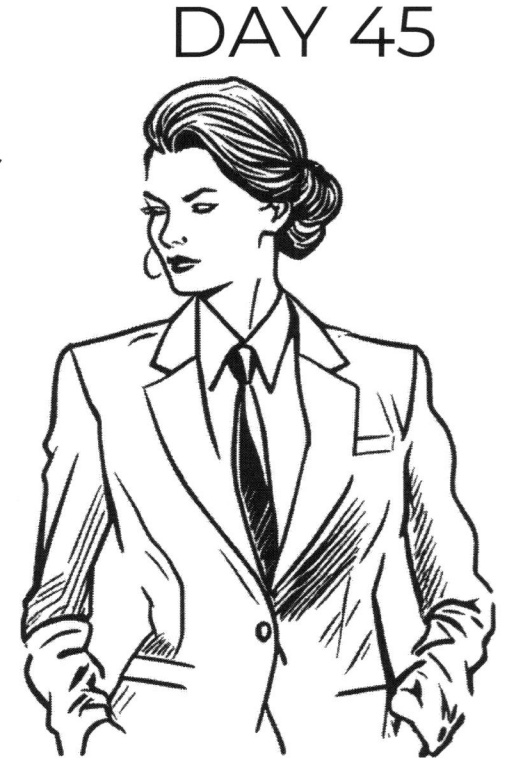

The Art of Becoming

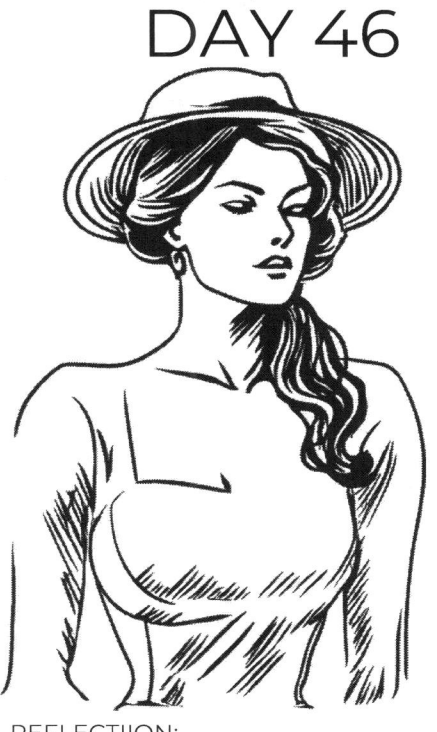

DAY 46

DAILY CHECK IN: ✓

- WOKE UP EARLY
- WENT TO THE GYM
- MORNING ROUTINE
- NIGHT ROUTINE
- ATE HEALTHY WHOLE FOODS
- READ AT LEAST 10 PAGES OF ANY BOOK

REFLECTIION:

_____
_____
_____
_____
_____
_____
_____
_____
_____

TODAY'S AFFIRMATION

MY ENERGY IS SACRED, AND I PROTECT IT FIERCELY

The Art of Becoming

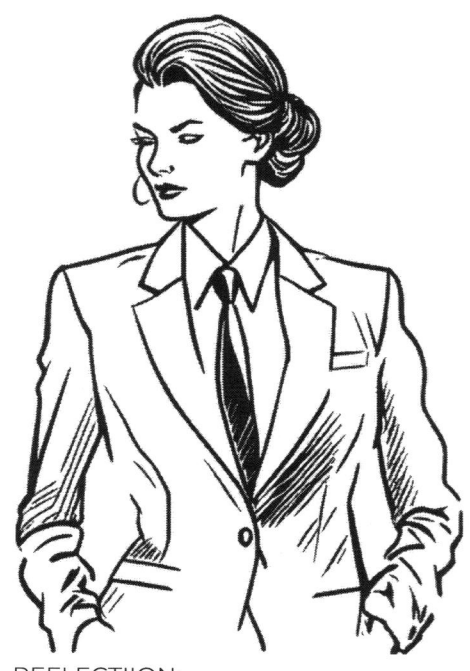

DAY 47

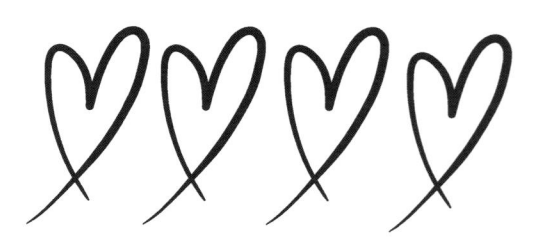

DAILY CHECK IN: ✓

- WOKE UP EARLY
- WENT TO THE GYM
- MORNING ROUTINE
- NIGHT ROUTINE
- ATE HEALTHY WHOLE FOODS
- READ AT LEAST 10 PAGES OF ANY BOOK

REFLECTIION:

_____
_____
_____
_____
_____
_____
_____
_____
_____
_____

TODAY'S AFFIRMATION

I LET GO OF COMPARISON AND CELEBRATE MY OWN JOURNEY

DAY 48

The Art of Becoming

DAILY CHECK IN: ✓

- WOKE UP EARLY
- WENT TO THE GYM
- MORNING ROUTINE
- NIGHT ROUTINE
- ATE HEALTHY WHOLE FOODS
- READ AT LEAST 10 PAGES OF ANY BOOK

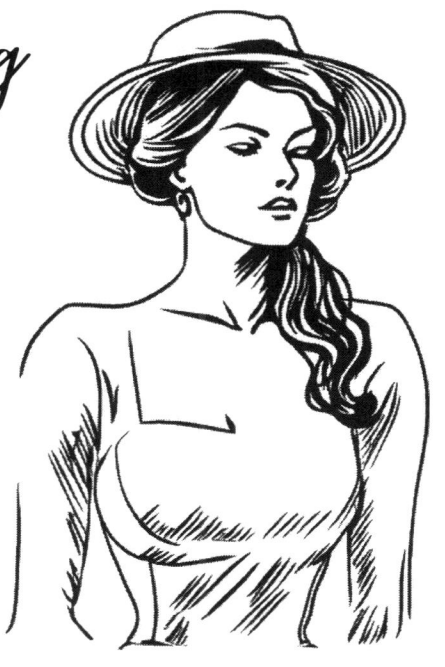

REFLECTIION:

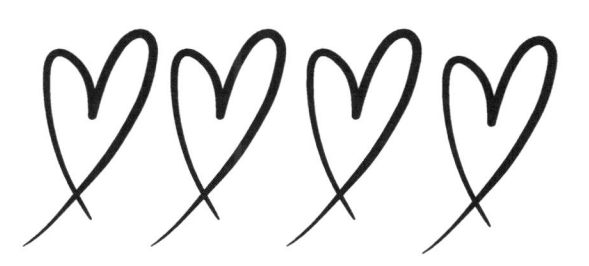

_____
_____
_____
_____
_____
_____
_____
_____
_____

TODAY'S AFFIRMATION

I EMBRACE SELF-CARE AS AN ACT OF SELF-LOVE

The Art of Becoming

DAY 49

DAILY CHECK IN: ✓

- WOKE UP EARLY ☐
- WENT TO THE GYM ☐
- MORNING ROUTINE ☐
- NIGHT ROUTINE ☐
- ATE HEALTHY WHOLE FOODS ☐
- READ AT LEAST 10 PAGES OF ANY BOOK ☐

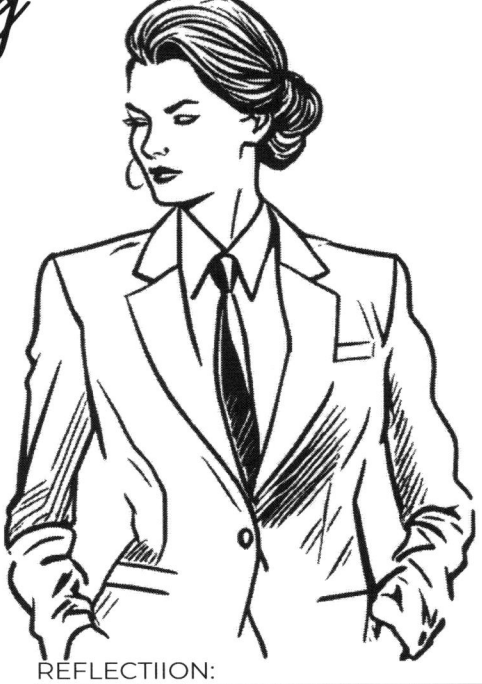

REFLECTIION:

_____
_____
_____
_____
_____
_____
_____
_____
_____

TODAY'S AFFIRMATION

I
TRUST
THAT I AM ENOUGH
JUST
AS I AM

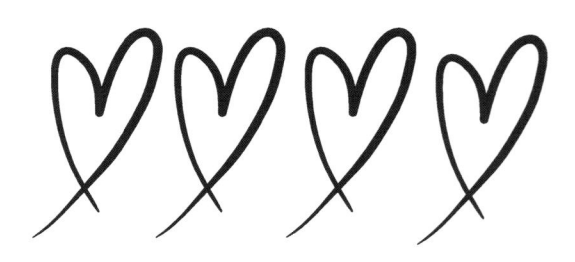

The Art of Becoming

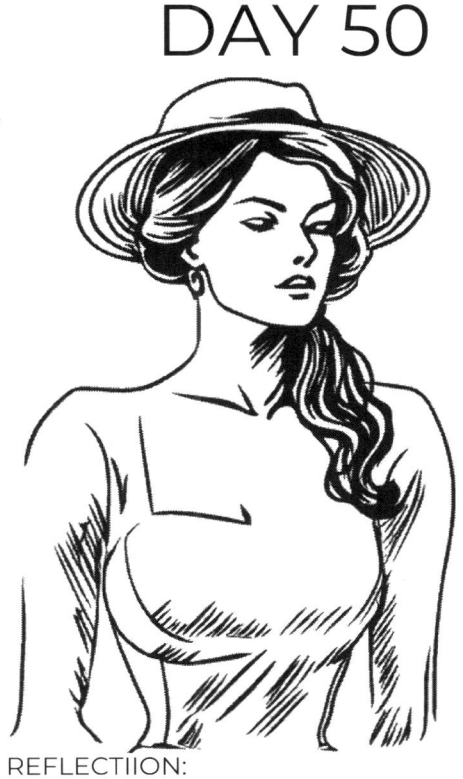

DAY 50

DAILY CHECK IN: ✓

- WOKE UP EARLY
- WENT TO THE GYM
- MORNING ROUTINE
- NIGHT ROUTINE
- ATE HEALTHY WHOLE FOODS
- READ AT LEAST 10 PAGES OF ANY BOOK

REFLECTIION:

_____
_____
_____
_____
_____
_____
_____
_____
_____

TODAY'S AFFIRMATION

I
AM
GLOWING FROM
THE
INSIDE OUT

The Art of Becoming

DAY 51

DAILY CHECK IN: ✓

- WOKE UP EARLY ☐
- WENT TO THE GYM ☐
- MORNING ROUTINE ☐
- NIGHT ROUTINE ☐
- ATE HEALTHY WHOLE FOODS ☐
- READ AT LEAST 10 PAGES OF ANY BOOK ☐

REFLECTIION:

_____
_____
_____
_____
_____
_____
_____
_____
_____

TODAY'S AFFIRMATION

I
GIVE MYSELF
GRACE
AS
I GROW

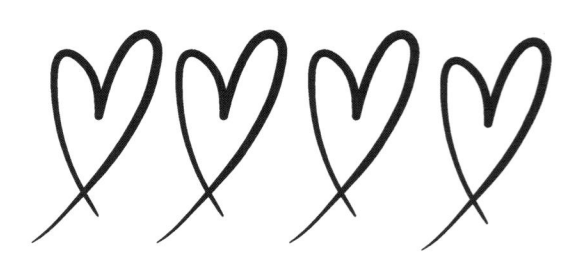

The Art of Becoming

DAY 52

DAILY CHECK IN: ✓

- WOKE UP EARLY
- WENT TO THE GYM
- MORNING ROUTINE
- NIGHT ROUTINE
- ATE HEALTHY WHOLE FOODS
- READ AT LEAST 10 PAGES OF ANY BOOK

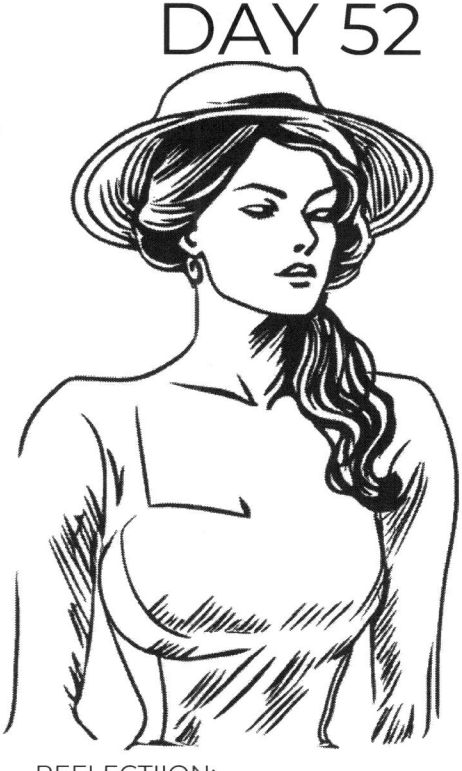

REFLECTIION:

_____
_____
_____
_____
_____
_____
_____
_____
_____

TODAY'S AFFIRMATION

I
DO NOT CHASE -
I ATTRACT
WHAT IS
MEANT FOR ME

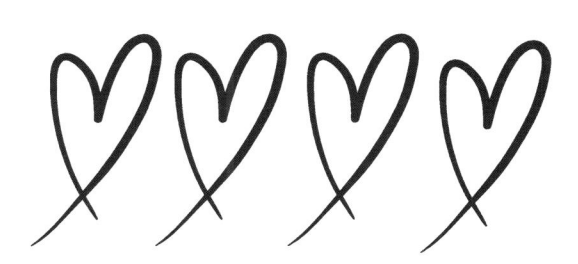

The Art of Becoming

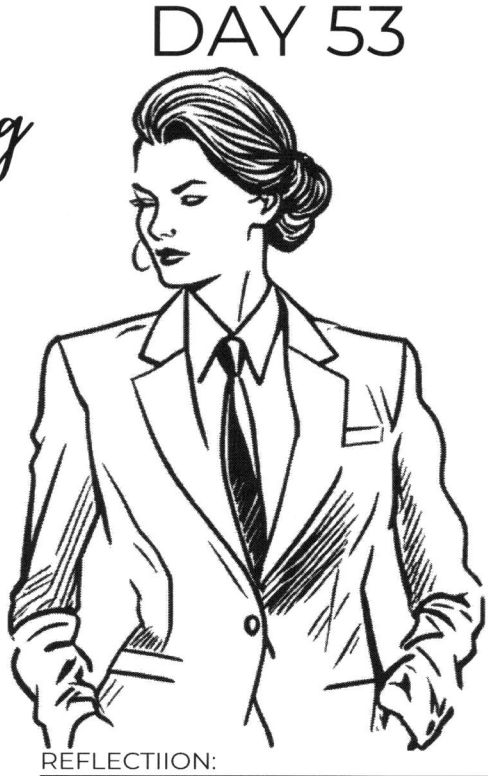

DAY 53

DAILY CHECK IN: ✓

- WOKE UP EARLY ☐
- WENT TO THE GYM ☐
- MORNING ROUTINE ☐
- NIGHT ROUTINE ☐
- ATE HEALTHY WHOLE FOODS ☐
- READ AT LEAST 10 PAGES OF ANY BOOK ☐

REFLECTIION:

_____
_____
_____
_____
_____
_____
_____
_____
_____
_____

TODAY'S AFFIRMATION

I
ONLY ENTERTAIN
RELATIONSHIPS THAT
UPLIFT
AND
HONOR ME

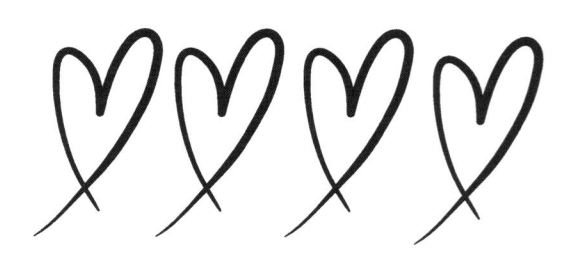

The Art of Becoming

DAY 54

DAILY CHECK IN: ✓ _____

- WOKE UP EARLY
- WENT TO THE GYM
- MORNING ROUTINE
- NIGHT ROUTINE
- ATE HEALTHY WHOLE FOODS
- READ AT LEAST 10 PAGES OF ANY BOOK

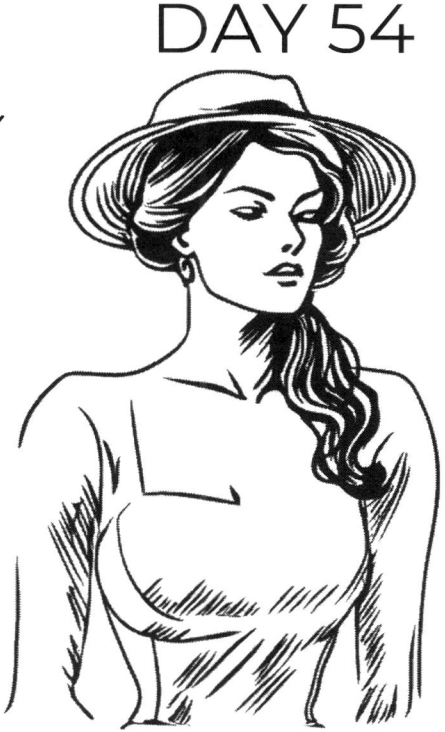

REFLECTIION: _____
_____
_____
_____
_____
_____
_____
_____
_____
_____

TODAY'S AFFIRMATION

I
AM GRATEFUL
FOR MY BODY
AND
ALL THAT IT DOES
FOR ME

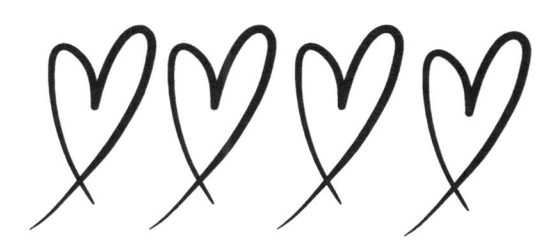

DAY 55

The Art of Becoming

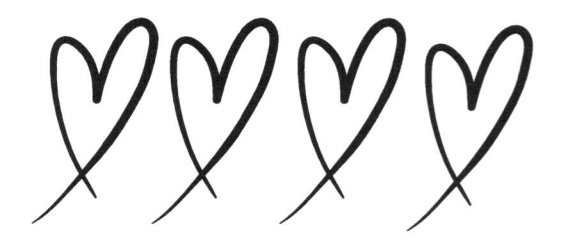

DAILY CHECK IN: ✓

- WOKE UP EARLY ☐
- WENT TO THE GYM ☐
- MORNING ROUTINE ☐
- NIGHT ROUTINE ☐
- ATE HEALTHY WHOLE FOODS ☐
- READ AT LEAST 10 PAGES OF ANY BOOK ☐

REFLECTIION: _____

_____
_____
_____
_____
_____
_____
_____
_____
_____

TODAY'S AFFIRMATION

MY SUCCESS IS BUILT ON DAILY HABITS, NOT JUST MOTIVATION

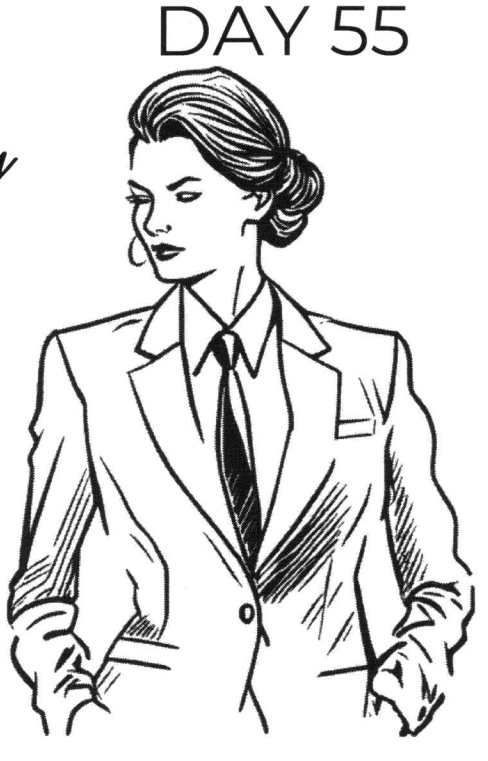

The Art of Becoming

DAY 56

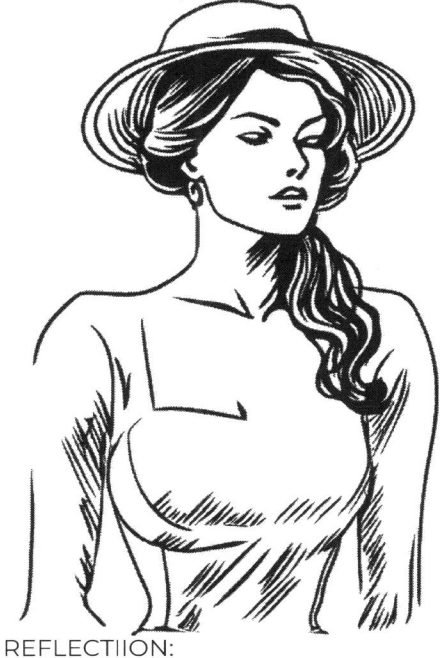

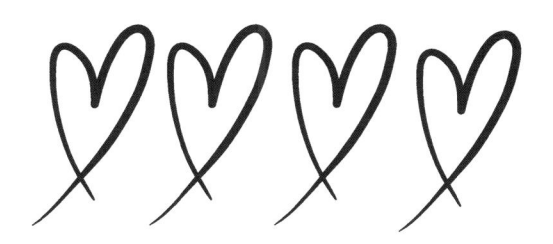

DAILY CHECK IN: ✓

- WOKE UP EARLY
- WENT TO THE GYM
- MORNING ROUTINE
- NIGHT ROUTINE
- ATE HEALTHY WHOLE FOODS
- READ AT LEAST 10 PAGES OF ANY BOOK

REFLECTIION:

_____
_____
_____
_____
_____
_____
_____
_____
_____

TODAY'S AFFIRMATION

I
SHOW UP
FOR
MYSELF EVEN WHEN
I
DON'T FEEL LIKE IT

The Art of Becoming

DAY 57

DAILY CHECK IN: ✓

- WOKE UP EARLY ☐
- WENT TO THE GYM ☐
- MORNING ROUTINE ☐
- NIGHT ROUTINE ☐
- ATE HEALTHY WHOLE FOODS ☐
- READ AT LEAST 10 PAGES OF ANY BOOK ☐

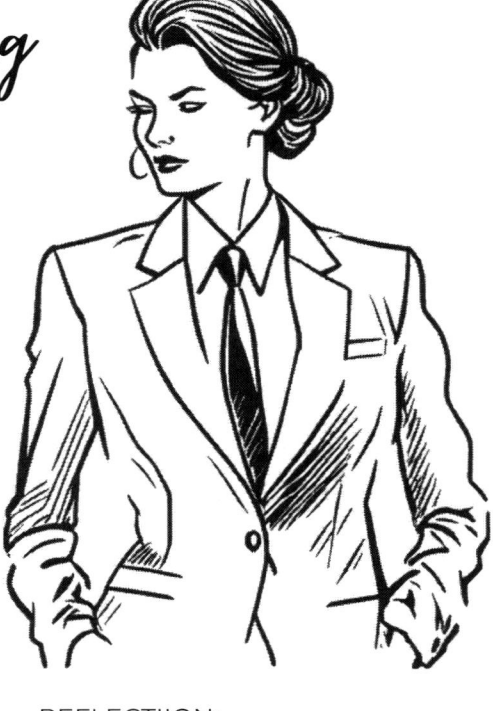

REFLECTIION:
_____
_____
_____
_____
_____
_____
_____
_____
_____

TODAY'S AFFIRMATION

SAME
DAILY
IMPROVEMENTS
LEAD TO MASSIVE
RESULTS
OVER TIME

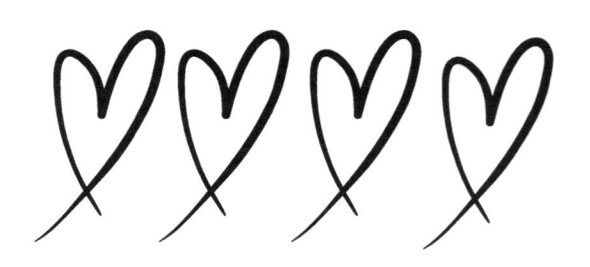

DAY 58

The Art of Becoming

DAILY CHECK IN: ✓

- WOKE UP EARLY
- WENT TO THE GYM
- MORNING ROUTINE
- NIGHT ROUTINE
- ATE HEALTHY WHOLE FOODS
- READ AT LEAST 10 PAGES OF ANY BOOK

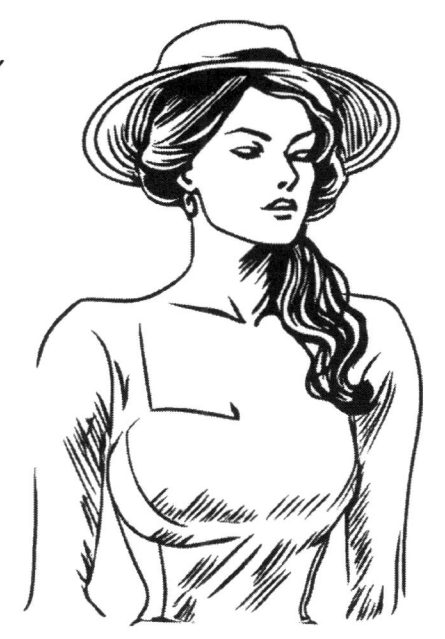

REFLECTIION:
_____
_____
_____
_____
_____
_____
_____
_____
_____

TODAY'S AFFIRMATION

I EMBRACE THE DISCIPLINE NEEDED TO BECOME MY HIGHEST SELF

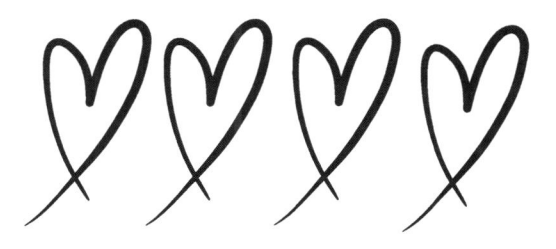

DAY 59

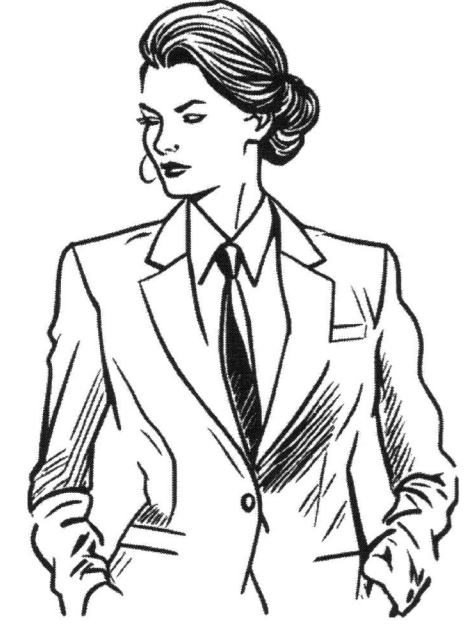

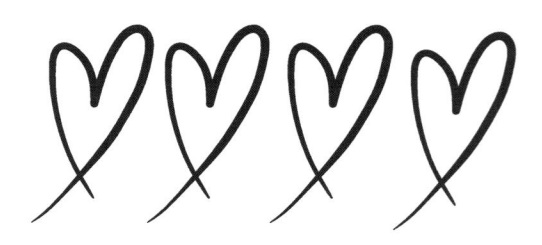

The Art of Becoming

DAILY CHECK IN: ✓

- WOKE UP EARLY ☐
- WENT TO THE GYM ☐
- MORNING ROUTINE ☐
- NIGHT ROUTINE ☐
- ATE HEALTHY WHOLE FOODS ☐
- READ AT LEAST 10 PAGES OF ANY BOOK ☐

REFLECTIION:

_____
_____
_____
_____
_____
_____
_____
_____
_____

TODAY'S AFFIRMATION

I STAY FOCUSED ON MY GOALS, KNOWING THAT CONSISTENCY IS KEY

DAY 60

The Art of Becoming

DAILY CHECK IN: ✓

- WOKE UP EARLY
- WENT TO THE GYM
- MORNING ROUTINE
- NIGHT ROUTINE
- ATE HEALTHY WHOLE FOODS
- READ AT LEAST 10 PAGES OF ANY BOOK

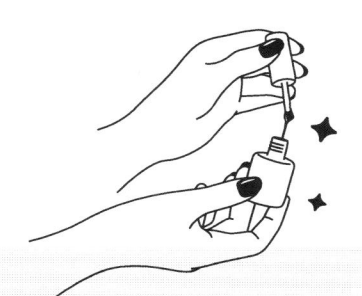

MAINTENANCE DAY TIME TO VISIT THE BEAUTY PARLOR BABES!

REFLECTIION:
_____
_____
_____
_____
_____
_____
_____
_____

TODAY'S AFFIRMATION

MY THOUGHTS CREATE MY REALITY - I CHOOSE TO THINK LIKE A WINNER

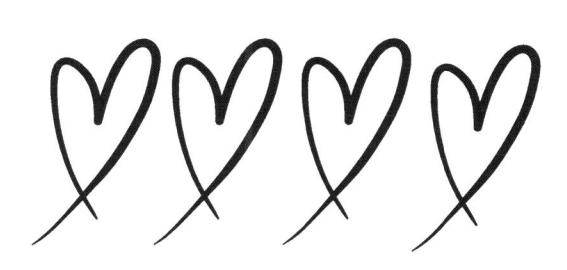

The Art of Becoming

DAY 61

DAILY CHECK IN: ✓

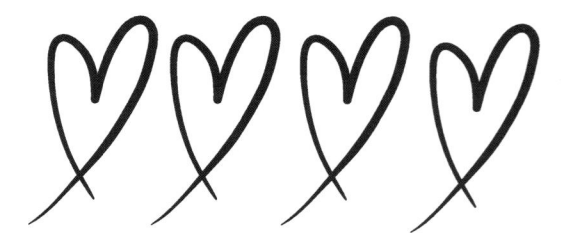

- WOKE UP EARLY
- WENT TO THE GYM
- MORNING ROUTINE
- NIGHT ROUTINE
- ATE HEALTHY WHOLE FOODS
- READ AT LEAST 10 PAGES OF ANY BOOK

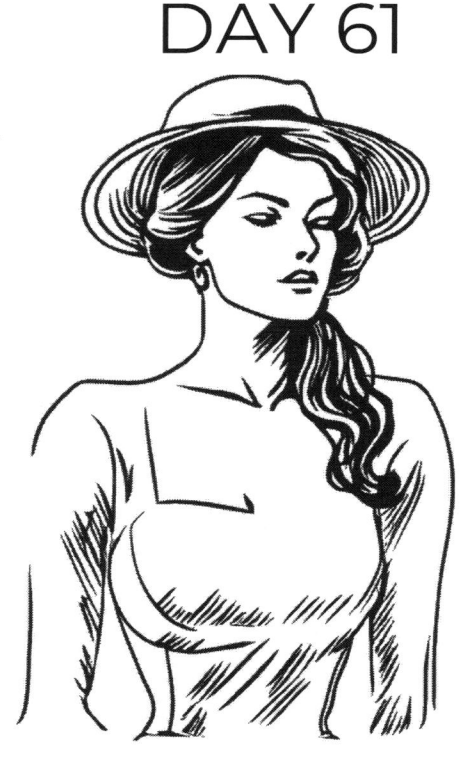

REFLECTIION:

_____
_____
_____
_____
_____
_____
_____
_____
_____

TODAY'S AFFIRMATION

I
RELEASE
PROCRASTINATION
AND TAKE ACTION
TOWARDS
MY
DREAM

The Art of Becoming

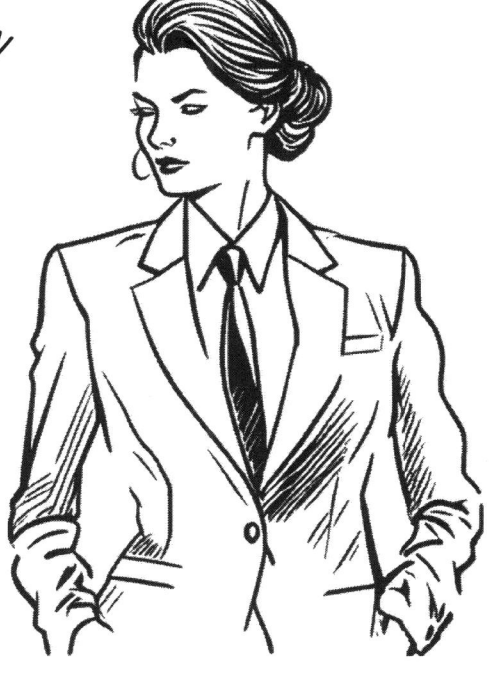

DAY 62

DAILY CHECK IN: ✓

- WOKE UP EARLY ☐
- WENT TO THE GYM ☐
- MORNING ROUTINE ☐
- NIGHT ROUTINE ☐
- ATE HEALTHY WHOLE FOODS ☐
- READ AT LEAST 10 PAGES OF ANY BOOK ☐

REFLECTIION:

_____
_____
_____
_____
_____
_____
_____
_____
_____

TODAY'S AFFIRMATION

I TRUST THE PROCESS, EVEN WHEN I DON'T SEE IMMEDIATE RESULTS

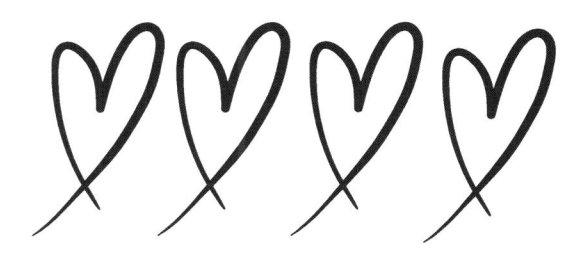

♡ ♡ ♡ ♡

The Art of Becoming

DAY 63

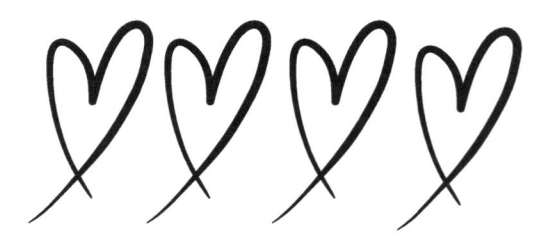

DAILY CHECK IN: ✓

- WOKE UP EARLY
- WENT TO THE GYM
- MORNING ROUTINE
- NIGHT ROUTINE
- ATE HEALTHY WHOLE FOODS
- READ AT LEAST 10 PAGES OF ANY BOOK

REFLECTIION:

_____
_____
_____
_____
_____
_____
_____
_____

TODAY'S AFFIRMATION

EVERY CHALLENGE I FACE STRENGHTENS MY MINDSET

The Art of Becoming

DAY 64

DAILY CHECK IN: ✓

- WOKE UP EARLY
- WENT TO THE GYM
- MORNING ROUTINE
- NIGHT ROUTINE
- ATE HEALTHY WHOLE FOODS
- READ AT LEAST 10 PAGES OF ANY BOOK

REFLECTIION:

_____
_____
_____
_____
_____
_____
_____
_____

TODAY'S AFFIRMATION

I AM IN CONTROL OF MY HABITS AND BUILD A LIFE THAT SUPPORTS MY SUCCESS

The Art of Becoming

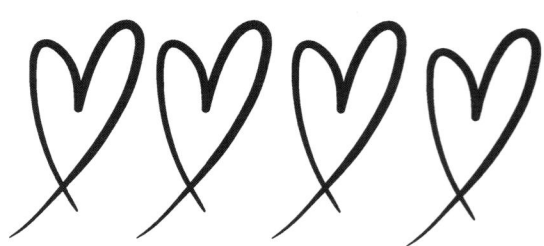

DAY 65

DAILY CHECK IN: ✓

- WOKE UP EARLY
- WENT TO THE GYM
- MORNING ROUTINE
- NIGHT ROUTINE
- ATE HEALTHY WHOLE FOODS
- READ AT LEAST 10 PAGES OF ANY BOOK

REFLECTIION:

_____
_____
_____
_____
_____
_____
_____
_____
_____

TODAY'S AFFIRMATION

I PRIORITIZE GROWTH OVER PERFECTION

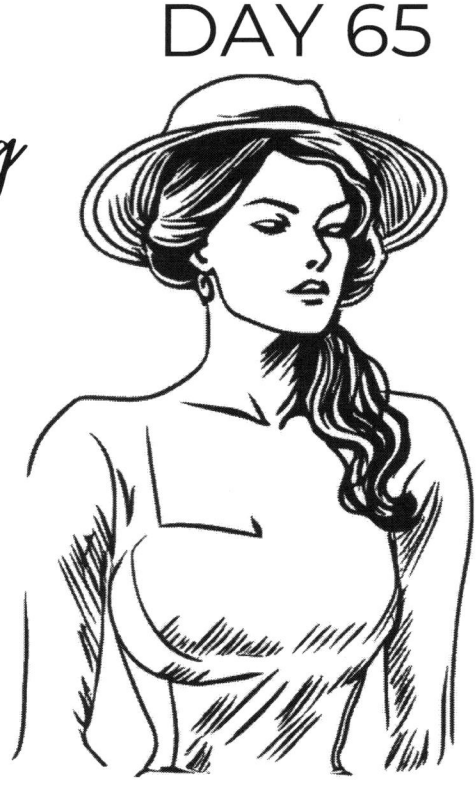

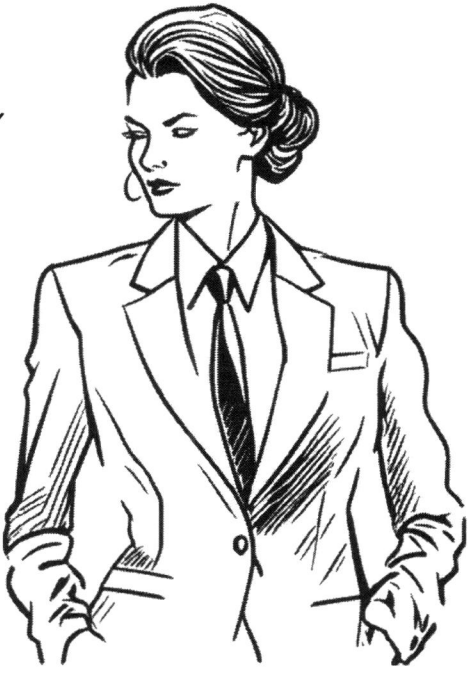

DAY 66

The Art of Becoming

DAILY CHECK IN: ✓

- WOKE UP EARLY
- WENT TO THE GYM
- MORNING ROUTINE
- NIGHT ROUTINE
- ATE HEALTHY WHOLE FOODS
- READ AT LEAST 10 PAGES OF ANY BOOK

REFLECTIION:

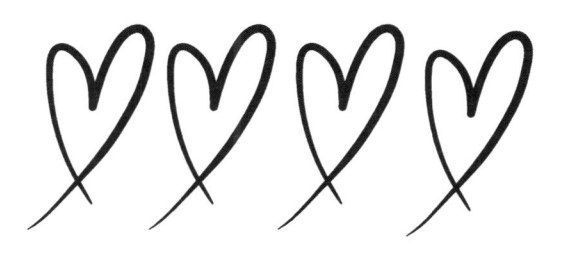

_____
_____
_____
_____
_____
_____
_____
_____
_____
_____

TODAY'S AFFIRMATION

I
SHOW UP
FOR MYSLEF,
EVEN
ON THE HARD DAYS

DAY 67

The Art of Becoming

DAILY CHECK IN: ✓

- WOKE UP EARLY
- WENT TO THE GYM
- MORNING ROUTINE
- NIGHT ROUTINE
- ATE HEALTHY WHOLE FOODS
- READ AT LEAST 10 PAGES OF ANY BOOK

REFLECTIION:

_____
_____
_____
_____
_____
_____
_____
_____
_____

TODAY'S AFFIRMATION

I
PUSH PAST MY
COMFORT ZONE
BECAUSE THAT IS
WHERE
GROWTH HAPPENS

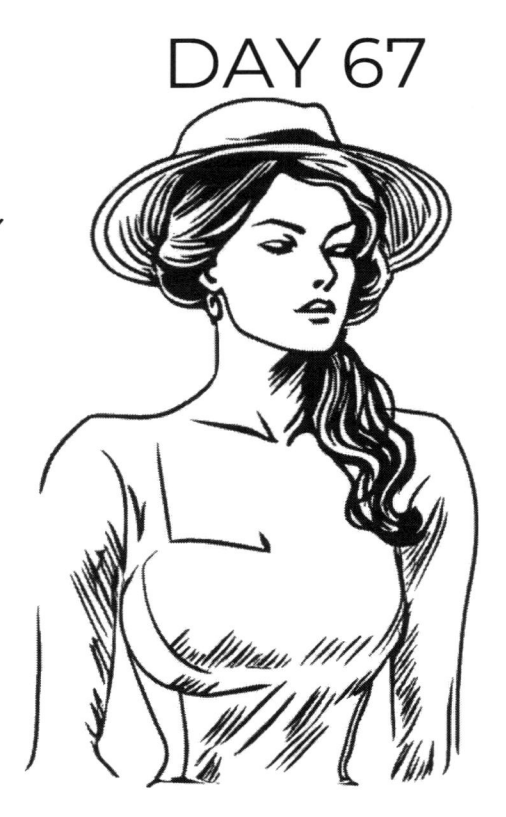

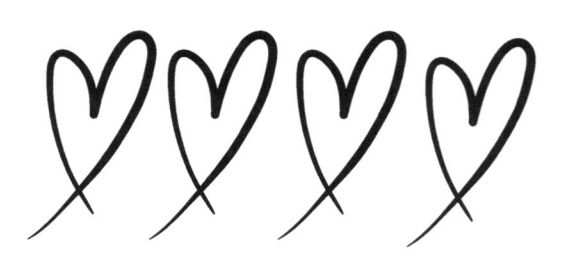

The Art of Becoming

DAY 68

DAILY CHECK IN: ✓

- WOKE UP EARLY ☐
- WENT TO THE GYM ☐
- MORNING ROUTINE ☐
- NIGHT ROUTINE ☐
- ATE HEALTHY WHOLE FOODS ☐
- READ AT LEAST 10 PAGES OF ANY BOOK ☐

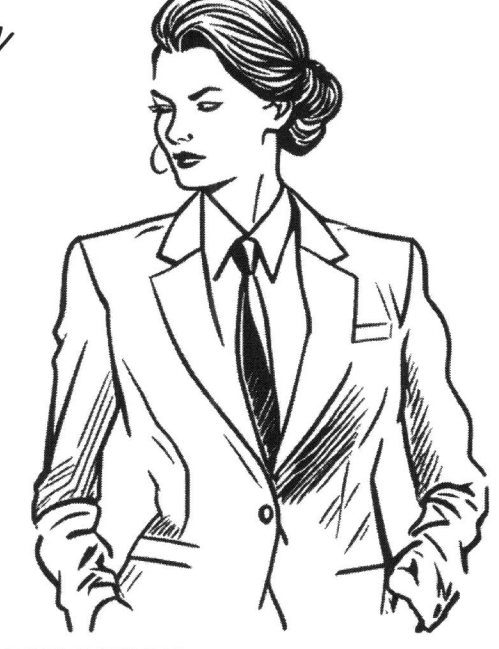

REFLECTIION:
_____
_____
_____
_____
_____
_____
_____
_____
_____
_____

TODAY'S AFFIRMATION

I FOLLOW THROUGH ON MY COMMITMENTS TO MYSELF

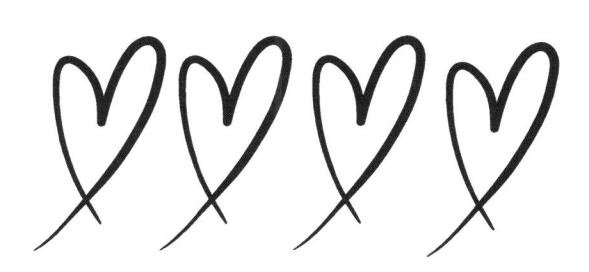

The Art of Becoming

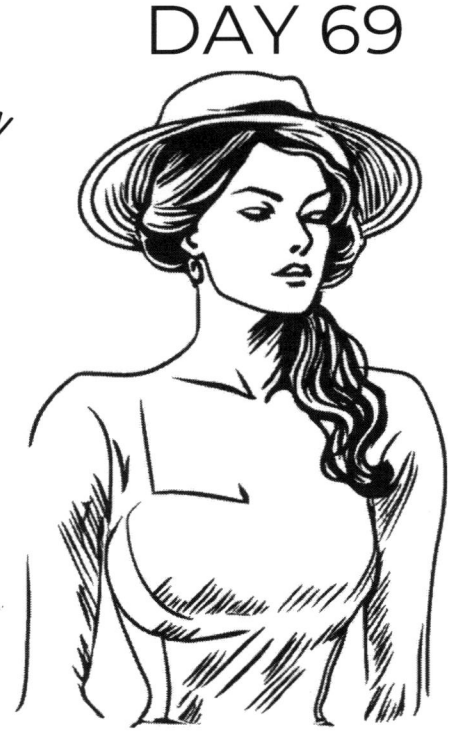

DAY 69

DAILY CHECK IN: ✓

- WOKE UP EARLY
- WENT TO THE GYM
- MORNING ROUTINE
- NIGHT ROUTINE
- ATE HEALTHY WHOLE FOODS
- READ AT LEAST 10 PAGES OF ANY BOOK

REFLECTIION:

_____
_____
_____
_____
_____
_____
_____
_____
_____

TODAY'S AFFIRMATION

I
TRUST MYSELF
TO
FIGURE THINGS
OUT
ALONG THE WAY

The Art of Becoming

DAY 70

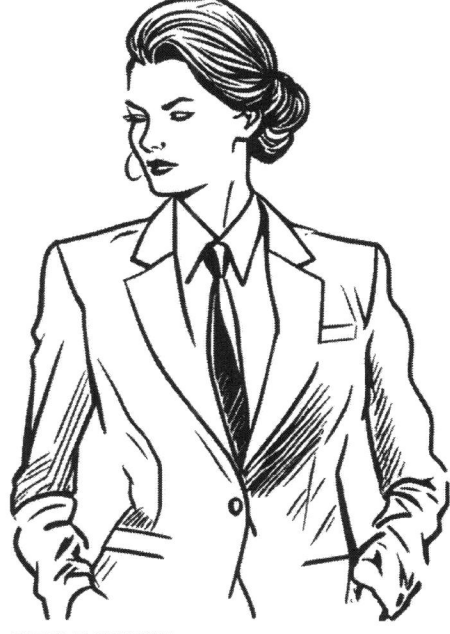

DAILY CHECK IN: ✓

- WOKE UP EARLY
- WENT TO THE GYM
- MORNING ROUTINE
- NIGHT ROUTINE
- ATE HEALTHY WHOLE FOODS
- READ AT LEAST 10 PAGES OF ANY BOOK

REFLECTIION:

_____
_____
_____
_____
_____
_____
_____
_____
_____

TODAY'S AFFIRMATION

I CELEBRATE PROGRESS, NO MATTER HOW SMALL

The Art of Becoming

DAY 71

DAILY CHECK IN: ✓

- WOKE UP EARLY
- WENT TO THE GYM
- MORNING ROUTINE
- NIGHT ROUTINE
- ATE HEALTHY WHOLE FOODS
- READ AT LEAST 10 PAGES OF ANY BOOK

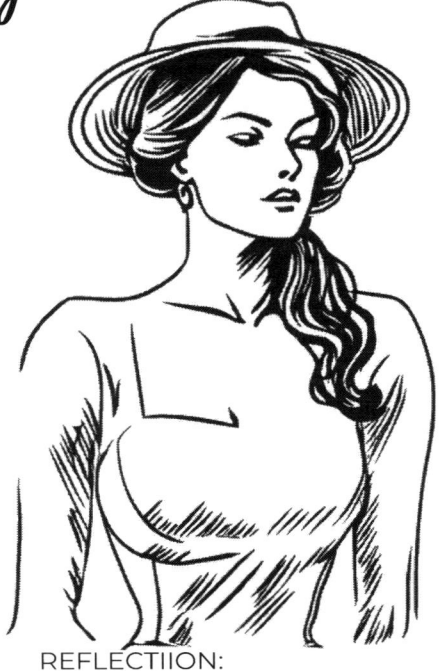

REFLECTIION:

_____
_____
_____
_____
_____
_____
_____
_____

TODAY'S AFFIRMATION

MY FUTURE SELF THANKS ME FOR THE EFFORT I PUT IN TODAY

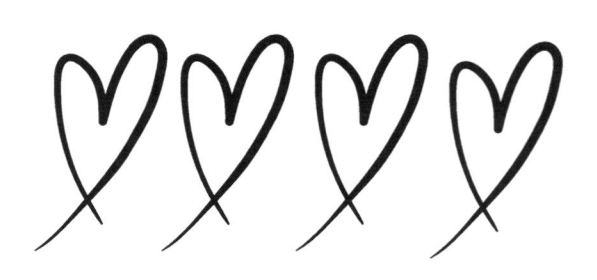

The Art of Becoming

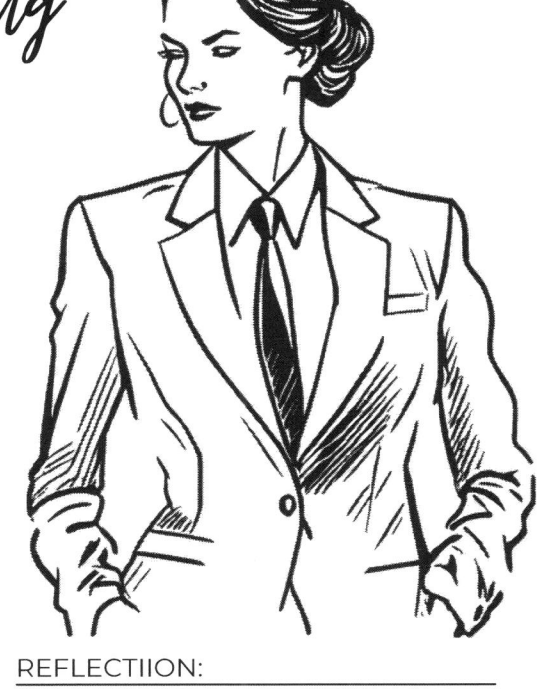

DAY 72

DAILY CHECK IN: ✓

- WOKE UP EARLY
- WENT TO THE GYM
- MORNING ROUTINE
- NIGHT ROUTINE
- ATE HEALTHY WHOLE FOODS
- READ AT LEAST 10 PAGES OF ANY BOOK

REFLECTIION:

_____
_____
_____
_____
_____
_____
_____
_____
_____

TODAY'S AFFIRMATION

I RELEASE ALL EXCUSES AND TAKE RESPONSIBILITY FOR MY SUCCESS

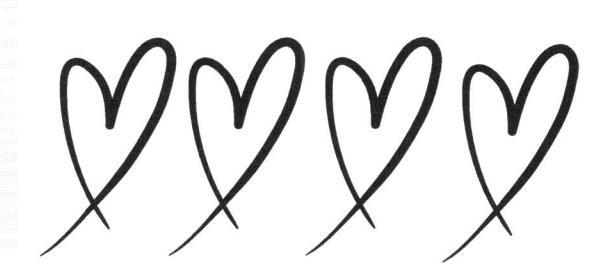

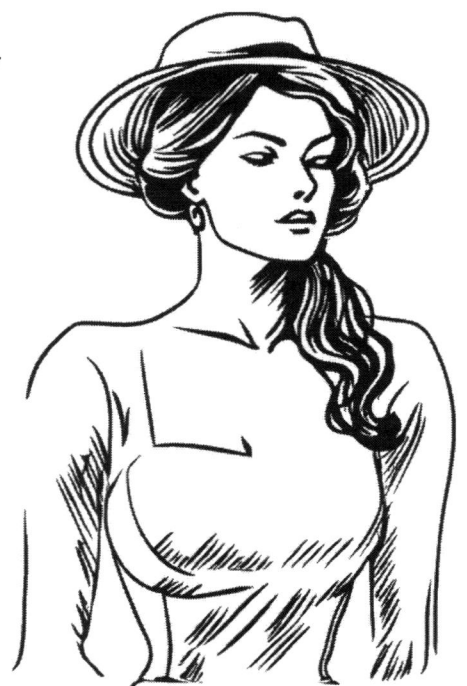

DAY 73

The Art of Becoming

DAILY CHECK IN: ✓

- WOKE UP EARLY
- WENT TO THE GYM
- MORNING ROUTINE
- NIGHT ROUTINE
- ATE HEALTHY WHOLE FOODS
- READ AT LEAST 10 PAGES OF ANY BOOK

REFLECTIION:

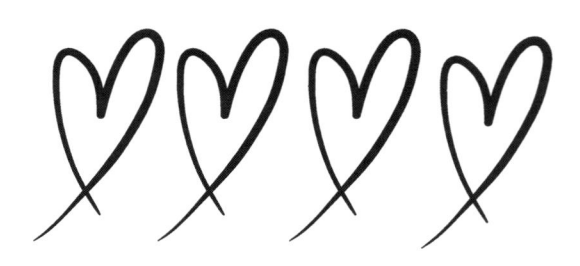

TODAY'S AFFIRMATION

I
BUILD
THE HABITS OF
THE
WOMAN I ASPIRE TO
BE

The Art of Becoming

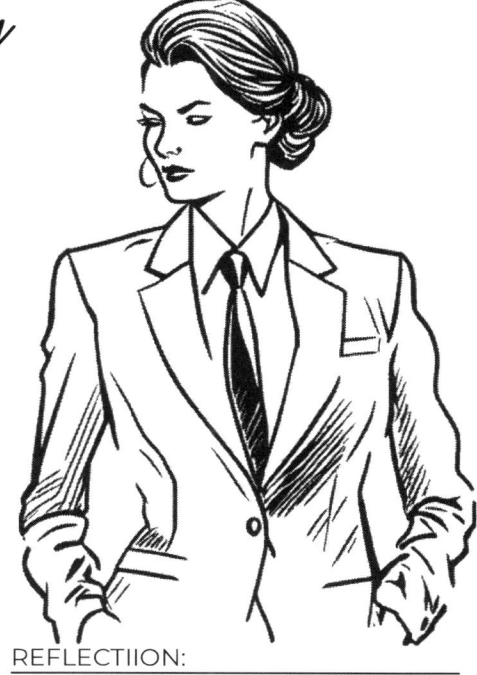

DAY 74

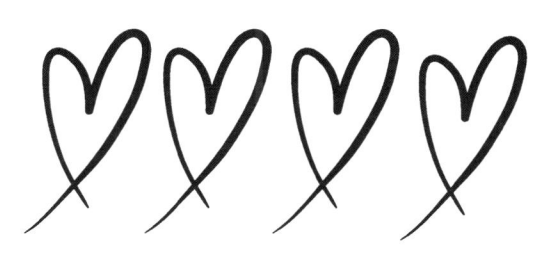

DAILY CHECK IN: ✓

- WOKE UP EARLY
- WENT TO THE GYM
- MORNING ROUTINE
- NIGHT ROUTINE
- ATE HEALTHY WHOLE FOODS
- READ AT LEAST 10 PAGES OF ANY BOOK

REFLECTIION:

_____
_____
_____
_____
_____
_____
_____
_____
_____
_____

TODAY'S AFFIRMATION

I INVEST IN MYSELF BECAUSE I AM MY GREATEST ASSET

The Art of Becoming

DAY 75

DAILY CHECK IN: ✓

- WOKE UP EARLY
- WENT TO THE GYM
- MORNING ROUTINE
- NIGHT ROUTINE
- ATE HEALTHY WHOLE FOODS
- READ AT LEAST 10 PAGES OF ANY BOOK

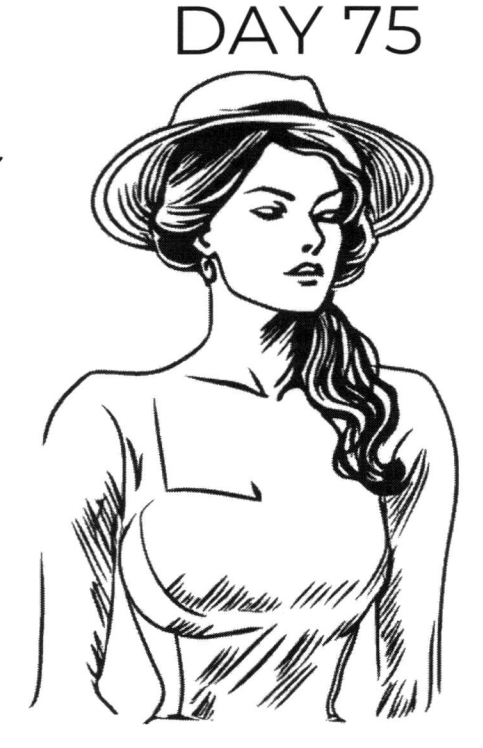

REFLECTIION:
_____
_____
_____
_____
_____
_____
_____
_____
_____

TODAY'S AFFIRMATION

I STAY COMMITTED TO MY GOALS, EVEN WHEN THE MOTIVATION FADES

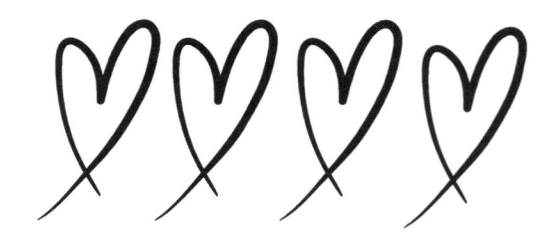

♡ ♡ ♡ ♡

The Art of Becoming

DAY 76

DAILY CHECK IN: ✓

- WOKE UP EARLY
- WENT TO THE GYM
- MORNING ROUTINE
- NIGHT ROUTINE
- ATE HEALTHY WHOLE FOODS
- READ AT LEAST 10 PAGES OF ANY BOOK

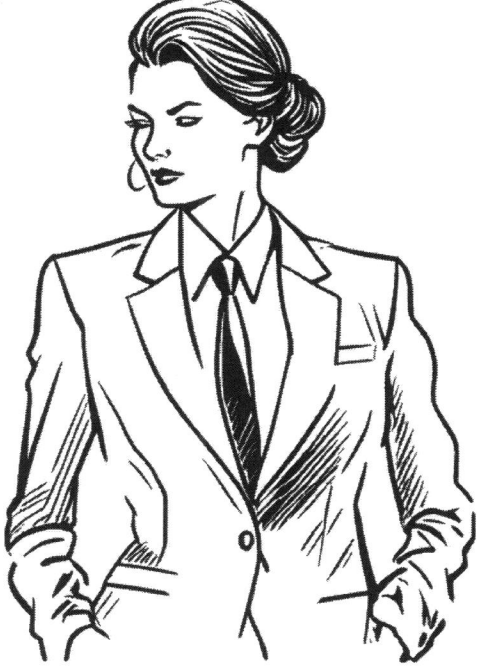

REFLECTIION:

_____
_____
_____
_____
_____
_____
_____
_____
_____

TODAY'S AFFIRMATION

I AM DEDICATED TO CREATING THE LIFE I DESIRE

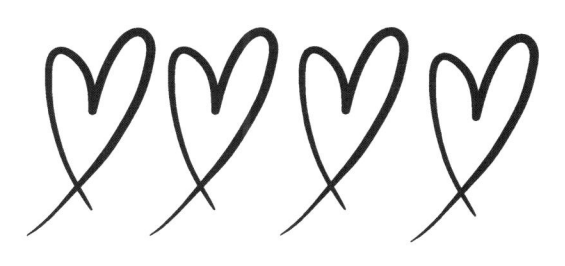

The Art of Becoming

DAY 77

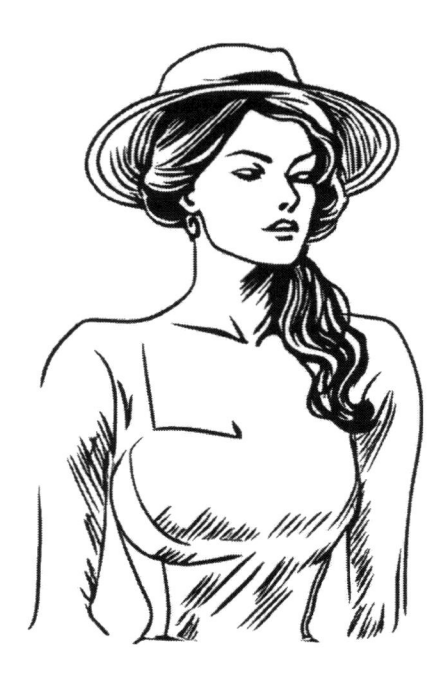

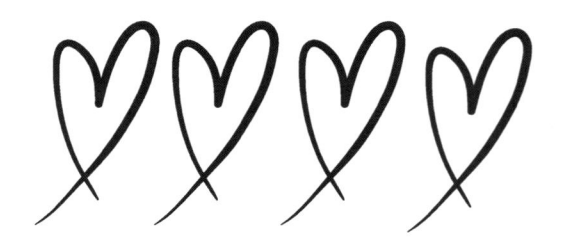

DAILY CHECK IN: ✓

- WOKE UP EARLY
- WENT TO THE GYM
- MORNING ROUTINE
- NIGHT ROUTINE
- ATE HEALTHY WHOLE FOODS
- READ AT LEAST 10 PAGES OF ANY BOOK

REFLECTIION:
_____
_____
_____
_____
_____
_____
_____
_____
_____

TODAY'S AFFIRMATION

I TRUST THE JOURNEY AND ENJOY THE PROCESS OF BECOMING MY BEST SELF

The Art of Becoming

DAY 78

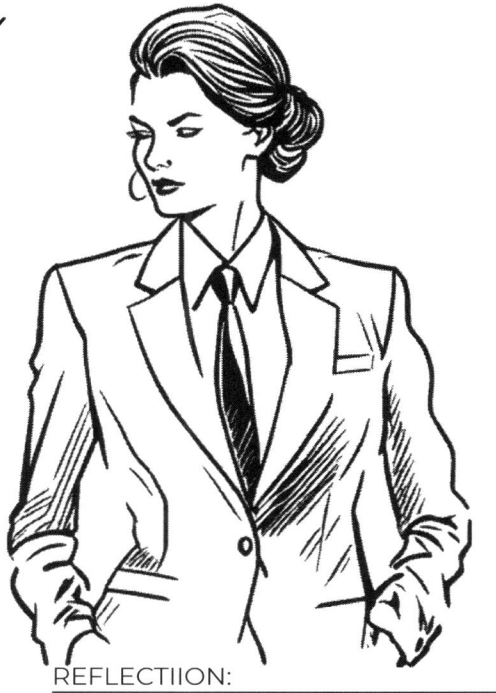

DAILY CHECK IN: ✓

- WOKE UP EARLY
- WENT TO THE GYM
- MORNING ROUTINE
- NIGHT ROUTINE
- ATE HEALTHY WHOLE FOODS
- READ AT LEAST 10 PAGES OF ANY BOOK

REFLECTIION:

_____
_____
_____
_____
_____
_____
_____
_____
_____

TODAY'S AFFIRMATION

MY
DAILY HABITS
SHAPE
THE LIFE
I AM
BUILDING

The Art of Becoming

DAY 79

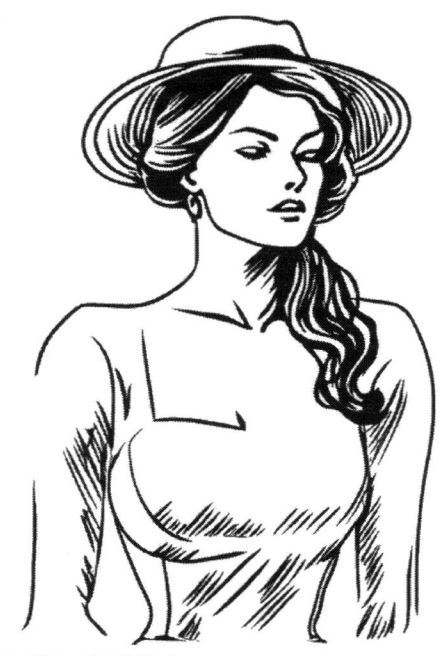

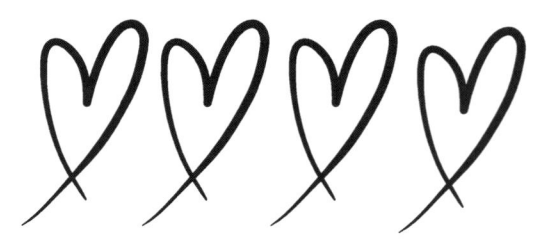

DAILY CHECK IN: ✓

- WOKE UP EARLY
- WENT TO THE GYM
- MORNING ROUTINE
- NIGHT ROUTINE
- ATE HEALTHY WHOLE FOODS
- READ AT LEAST 10 PAGES OF ANY BOOK

REFLECTIION:
_____
_____
_____
_____
_____
_____
_____
_____
_____

TODAY'S AFFIRMATION

I EMBODY DISCIPLINE AND CONSISTENCY NEEDED TO SUCCEED

The Art of Becoming

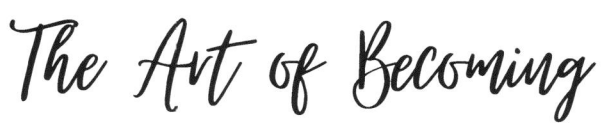

DAY 80

DAILY CHECK IN: ✓

- WOKE UP EARLY
- WENT TO THE GYM
- MORNING ROUTINE
- NIGHT ROUTINE
- ATE HEALTHY WHOLE FOODS
- READ AT LEAST 10 PAGES OF ANY BOOK

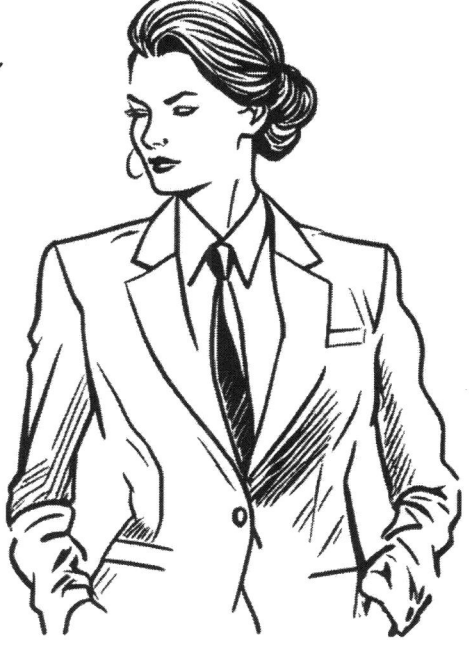

REFLECTIION:
_____
_____
_____
_____
_____
_____
_____
_____
_____

TODAY'S AFFIRMATION

MY SOFTNESS IS MY STRENGTH, NOT A WEAKNESS

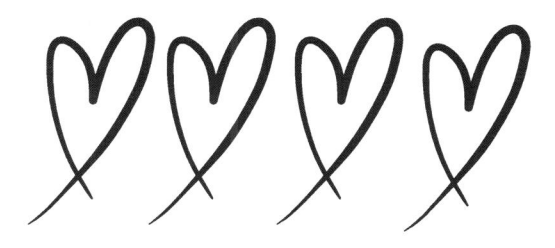

The Art of Becoming

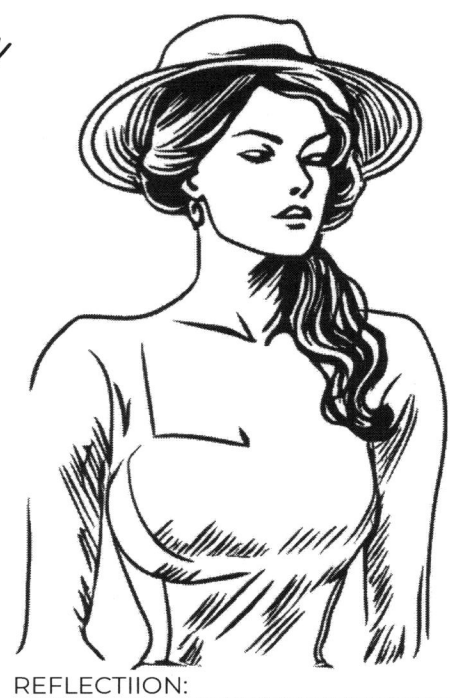

DAY 81

DAILY CHECK IN: ✓

- WOKE UP EARLY
- WENT TO THE GYM
- MORNING ROUTINE
- NIGHT ROUTINE
- ATE HEALTHY WHOLE FOODS
- READ AT LEAST 10 PAGES OF ANY BOOK

REFLECTIION:

_____
_____
_____
_____
_____
_____
_____
_____
_____

TODAY'S AFFIRMATION

I RADIATE WARMTH, KINDNESS, AND ELEGANCE IN ALL THAT I DO

The Art of Becoming

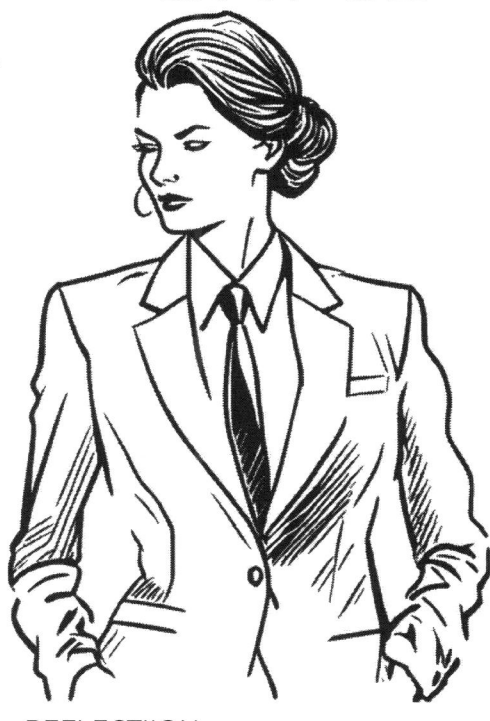

DAY 82

DAILY CHECK IN: ✓

- WOKE UP EARLY
- WENT TO THE GYM
- MORNING ROUTINE
- NIGHT ROUTINE
- ATE HEALTHY WHOLE FOODS
- READ AT LEAST 10 PAGES OF ANY BOOK

REFLECTIION:

_____
_____
_____
_____
_____
_____
_____
_____

TODAY'S AFFIRMATION

I NURTURE MYSELF AND HONOR MY EMOTIONS

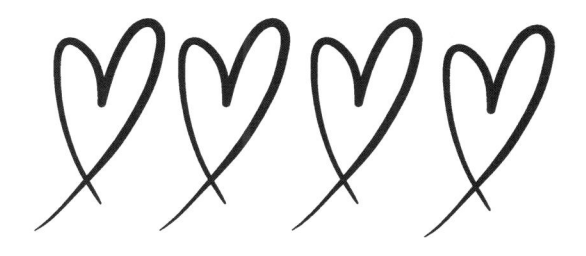

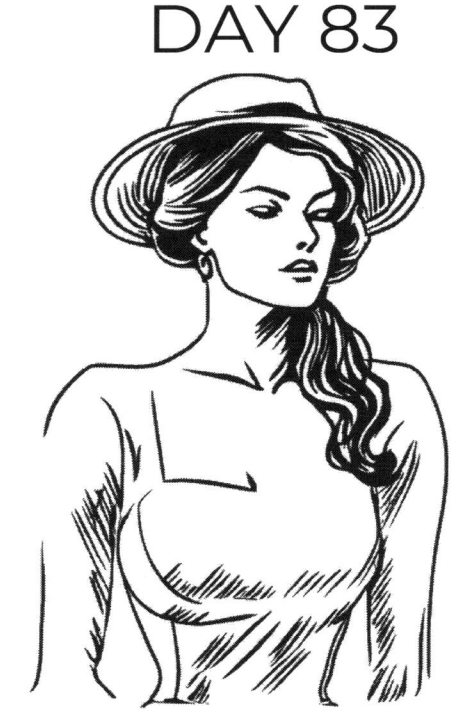

The Art of Becoming

DAY 83

DAILY CHECK IN: ✓

- WOKE UP EARLY ☐
- WENT TO THE GYM ☐
- MORNING ROUTINE ☐
- NIGHT ROUTINE ☐
- ATE HEALTHY WHOLE FOODS ☐
- READ AT LEAST 10 PAGES OF ANY BOOK ☐

REFLECTIION:

_____
_____
_____
_____
_____
_____
_____
_____

TODAY'S AFFIRMATION

I LET GO THE NEED TO CONTROL AND SURRENDER TO DIVINE TIMING

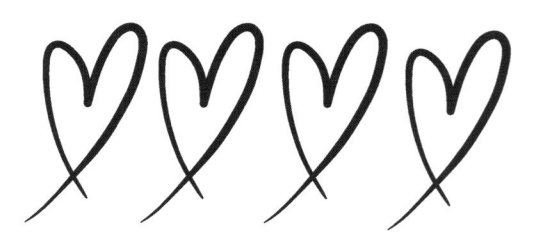

DAY 84

The Art of Becoming

DAILY CHECK IN: ✓

- WOKE UP EARLY
- WENT TO THE GYM
- MORNING ROUTINE
- NIGHT ROUTINE
- ATE HEALTHY WHOLE FOODS
- READ AT LEAST 10 PAGES OF ANY BOOK

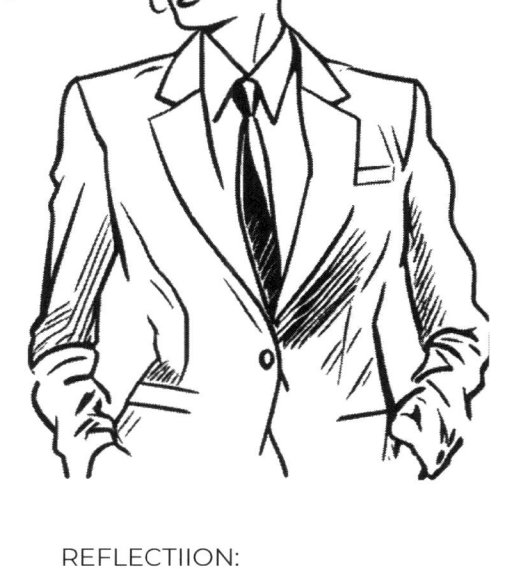

REFLECTIION:

_____
_____
_____
_____
_____
_____
_____
_____

TODAY'S AFFIRMATION

I ALLOW LIFE TO UNFOLD BEAUTIFULLY, KNOWING EVERYTHING IS WORKING IN MY FAVOR

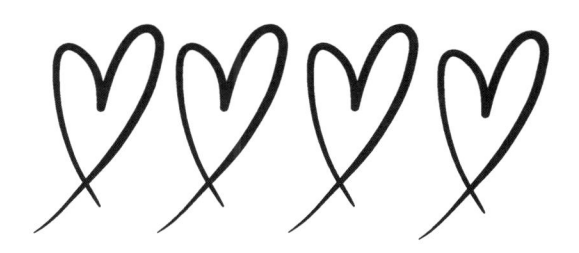

DAY 85

The Art of Becoming

DAILY CHECK IN: ✓

- WOKE UP EARLY
- WENT TO THE GYM
- MORNING ROUTINE
- NIGHT ROUTINE
- ATE HEALTHY WHOLE FOODS
- READ AT LEAST 10 PAGES OF ANY BOOK

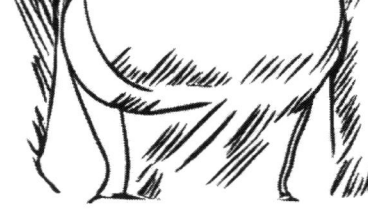

REFLECTIION:
_____
_____
_____
_____
_____
_____
_____
_____
_____

TODAY'S AFFIRMATION

I
LEAN INTO MY
SOFTNESS
AND
EMBRACE MY
NURTURING NATURE

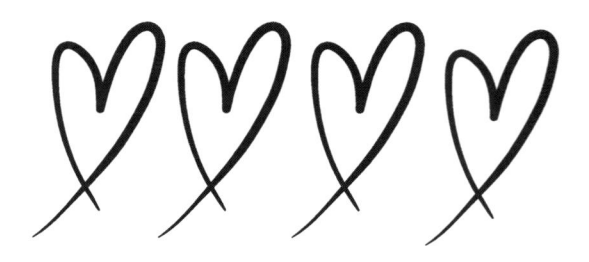

The Art of Becoming

DAY 86

DAILY CHECK IN: ✓

- WOKE UP EARLY
- WENT TO THE GYM
- MORNING ROUTINE
- NIGHT ROUTINE
- ATE HEALTHY WHOLE FOODS
- READ AT LEAST 10 PAGES OF ANY BOOK

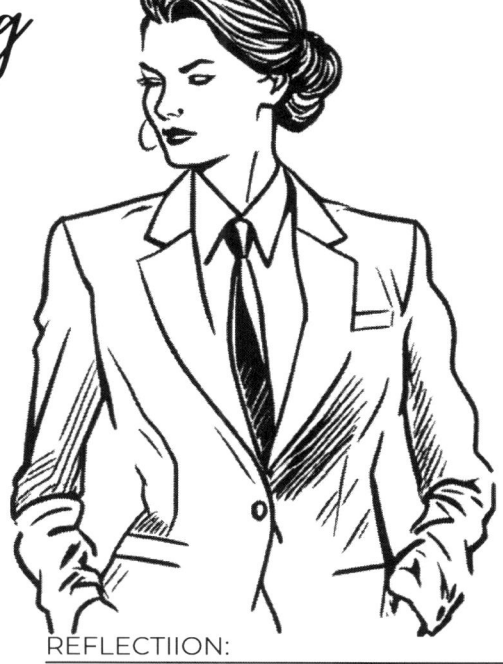

REFLECTIION:

_____
_____
_____
_____
_____
_____
_____
_____
_____

TODAY'S AFFIRMATION

I LET GO OF STRUGGLING AND EMBRACE THE ART OF ALLOWING

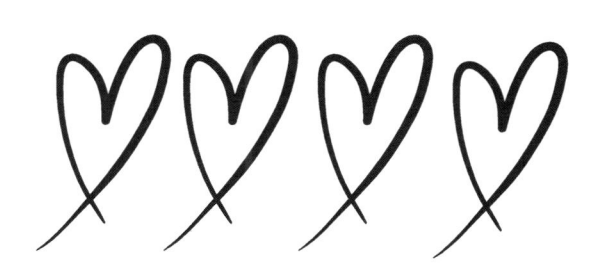

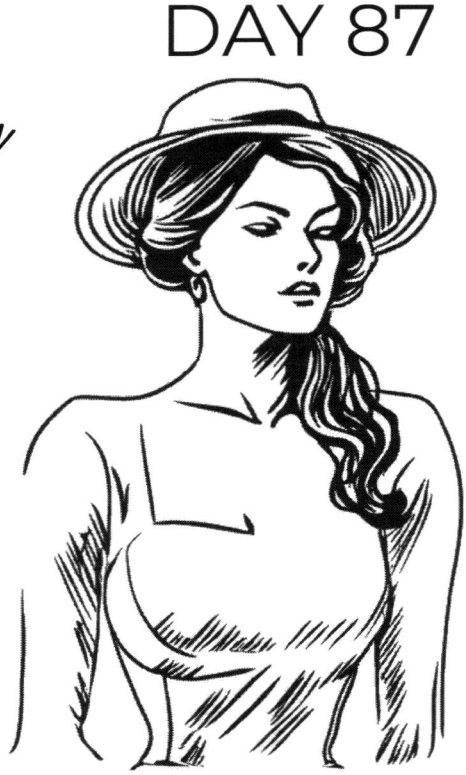

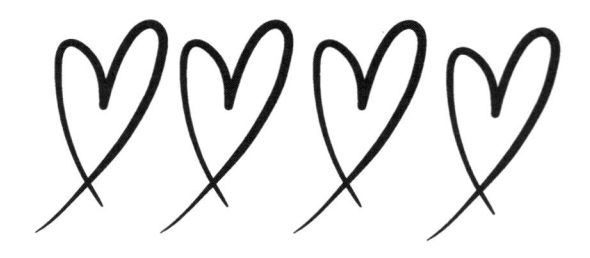

The Art of Becoming

DAY 87

DAILY CHECK IN: ✓

- WOKE UP EARLY ☐
- WENT TO THE GYM ☐
- MORNING ROUTINE ☐
- NIGHT ROUTINE ☐
- ATE HEALTHY WHOLE FOODS ☐
- READ AT LEAST 10 PAGES OF ANY BOOK ☐

REFLECTIION:

_____
_____
_____
_____
_____
_____
_____
_____
_____

TODAY'S AFFIRMATION

MY FEMININITY IS POWERFUL, AND I EXPRESS IT WITH PRIDE

The Art of Becoming

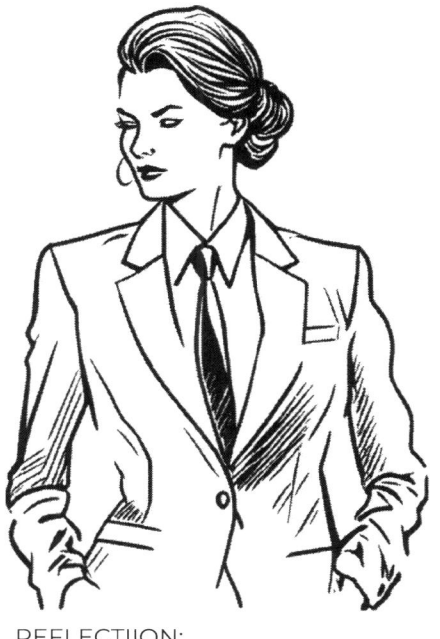

DAY 88

DAILY CHECK IN: ✓

- WOKE UP EARLY
- WENT TO THE GYM
- MORNING ROUTINE
- NIGHT ROUTINE
- ATE HEALTHY WHOLE FOODS
- READ AT LEAST 10 PAGES OF ANY BOOK

REFLECTIION:

_____
_____
_____
_____
_____
_____
_____
_____
_____

TODAY'S AFFIRMATION

THE WAY I DRESS REFLECTS THE POWERFUL WOMAN I AM BECOMING

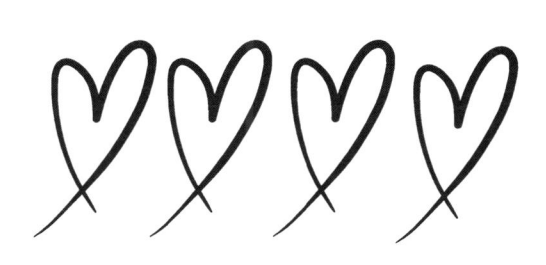

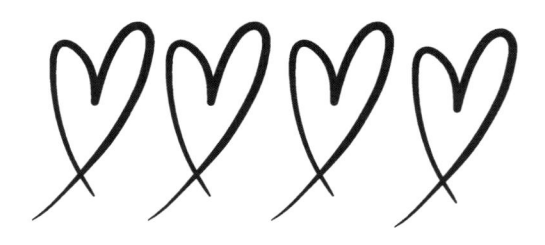

The Art of Becoming

DAY 89

DAILY CHECK IN: ✓

- WOKE UP EARLY
- WENT TO THE GYM
- MORNING ROUTINE
- NIGHT ROUTINE
- ATE HEALTHY WHOLE FOODS
- READ AT LEAST 10 PAGES OF ANY BOOK

REFLECTIION:

_____
_____
_____
_____
_____
_____
_____
_____
_____

TODAY'S AFFIRMATION

I DRESS IN A WAY THAT ELEVATES MY SELF-IMAGE

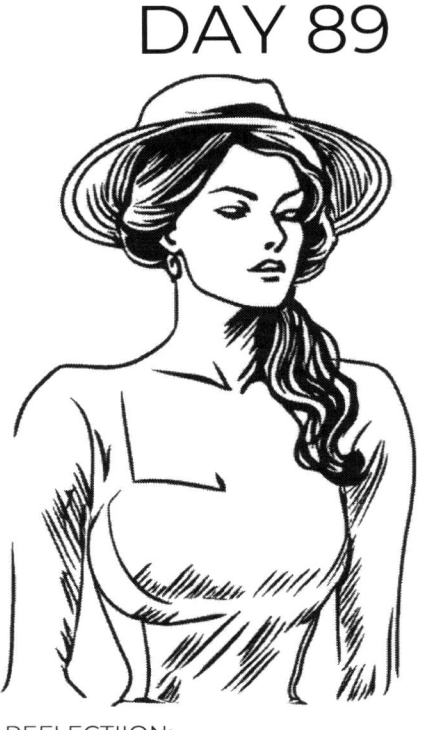

DAY 90

The Art of Becoming

DAILY CHECK IN: ✓

- WOKE UP EARLY
- WENT TO THE GYM
- MORNING ROUTINE
- NIGHT ROUTINE
- ATE HEALTHY WHOLE FOODS
- READ AT LEAST 10 PAGES OF ANY BOOK

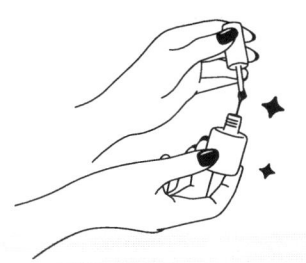

MAINTENANCE DAY
TIME
TO VISIT THE
BEAUTY PARLOR
BABES!

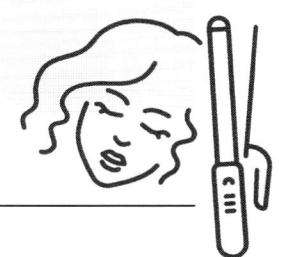

REFLECTIION:
_____
_____
_____

_____
_____
_____
_____
_____
_____

TODAY'S AFFIRMATION

MY PERSONAL STYLE IS AN EXTENSION OF MY IDENTITY

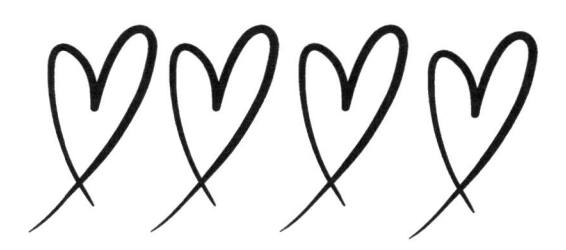

DAY 91

The Art of Becoming

DAILY CHECK IN: ✓

- WOKE UP EARLY
- WENT TO THE GYM
- MORNING ROUTINE
- NIGHT ROUTINE
- ATE HEALTHY WHOLE FOODS
- READ AT LEAST 10 PAGES OF ANY BOOK

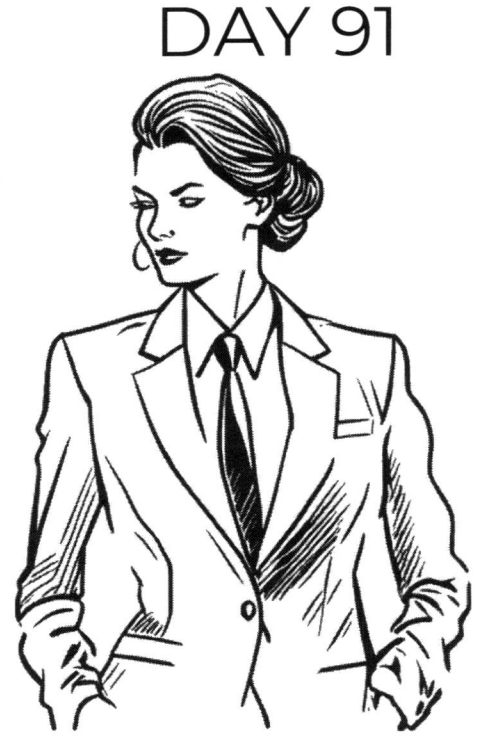

REFLECTIION:
_____
_____
_____
_____
_____
_____
_____
_____
_____
_____

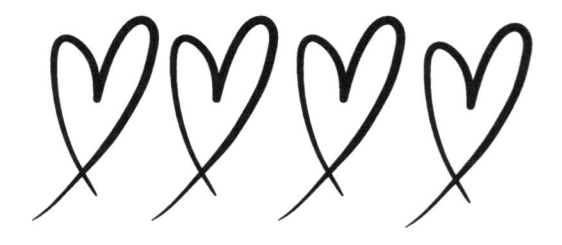

TODAY'S AFFIRMATION

I PRESENT MYSELF WITH ELEGANCE AND INTENTION

The Art of Becoming

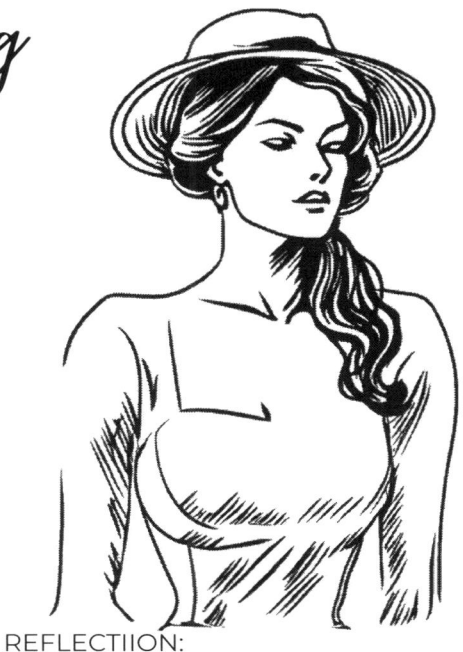

DAY 92

DAILY CHECK IN: ✓

- WOKE UP EARLY
- WENT TO THE GYM
- MORNING ROUTINE
- NIGHT ROUTINE
- ATE HEALTHY WHOLE FOODS
- READ AT LEAST 10 PAGES OF ANY BOOK

REFLECTIION:

_____
_____
_____
_____
_____
_____
_____
_____

TODAY'S AFFIRMATION

I
AM
COMMITTED TO MY
HEALTH
AND
WELL-BEING

DAY 93

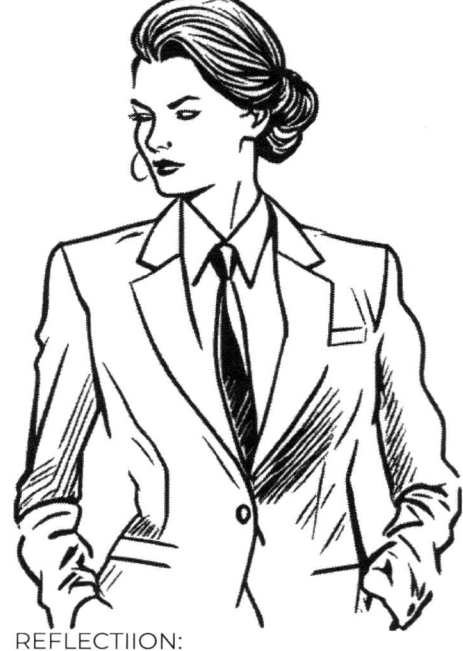

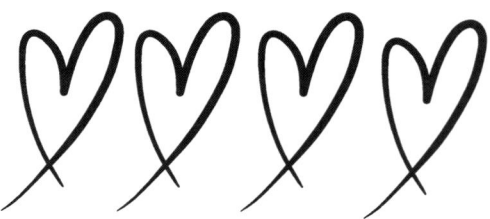

The Art of Becoming

DAILY CHECK IN: ✓

- WOKE UP EARLY
- WENT TO THE GYM
- MORNING ROUTINE
- NIGHT ROUTINE
- ATE HEALTHY WHOLE FOODS
- READ AT LEAST 10 PAGES OF ANY BOOK

REFLECTIION:

_____
_____
_____
_____
_____
_____
_____
_____
_____

TODAY'S AFFIRMATION

I RADIATE HEALTH, VIBRANCY, AND BEAUTY EFFORTLESSLY

DAY 94

The Art of Becoming

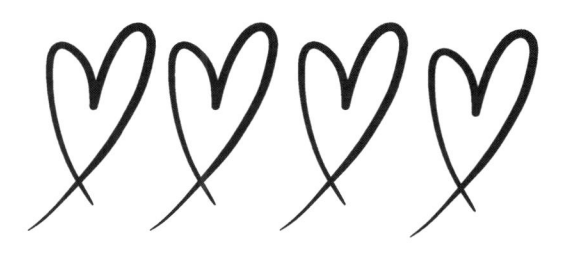

DAILY CHECK IN: ✓

- WOKE UP EARLY
- WENT TO THE GYM
- MORNING ROUTINE
- NIGHT ROUTINE
- ATE HEALTHY WHOLE FOODS
- READ AT LEAST 10 PAGES OF ANY BOOK

REFLECTIION:

TODAY'S AFFIRMATION

I RELEASE TOXIC RELATIONSHIPS AND CHOOSE HEALTHY CONNECTIONS

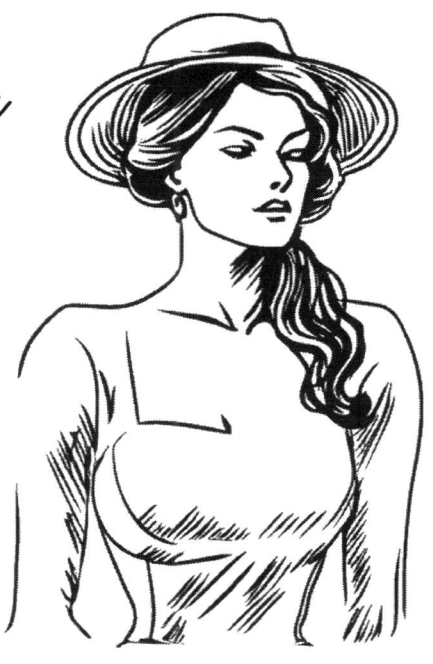

The Art of Becoming

DAY 95

DAILY CHECK IN: ✓

- WOKE UP EARLY ☐
- WENT TO THE GYM ☐
- MORNING ROUTINE ☐
- NIGHT ROUTINE ☐
- ATE HEALTHY WHOLE FOODS ☐
- READ AT LEAST 10 PAGES OF ANY BOOK ☐

REFLECTIION:

_____
_____
_____
_____
_____
_____
_____
_____
_____

TODAY'S AFFIRMATION

I AM CONFIDENT IN SAYING NO TO THINGS THAT DON'T SERVE ME

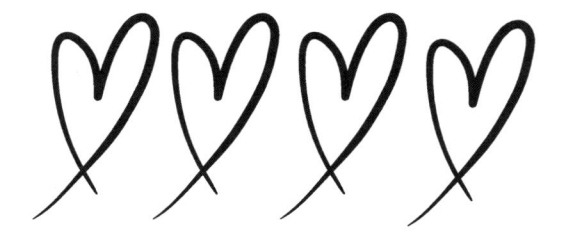

The Art of Becoming

DAY 96

DAILY CHECK IN: ✓

- WOKE UP EARLY
- WENT TO THE GYM
- MORNING ROUTINE
- NIGHT ROUTINE
- ATE HEALTHY WHOLE FOODS
- READ AT LEAST 10 PAGES OF ANY BOOK

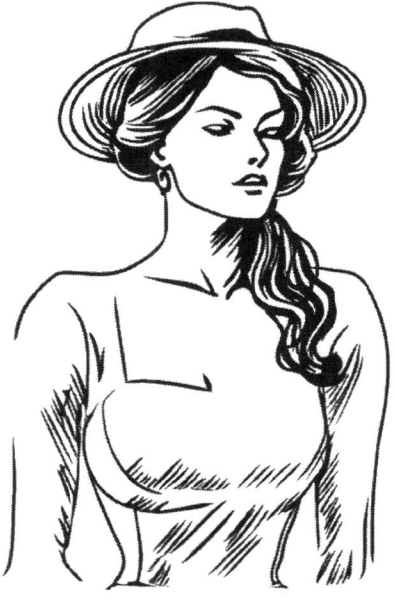

REFLECTIION:

_____
_____
_____
_____
_____
_____
_____
_____
_____

TODAY'S AFFIRMATION

I SET BOUNDARIES TO PROTECT MY ENERGY AND PEACE

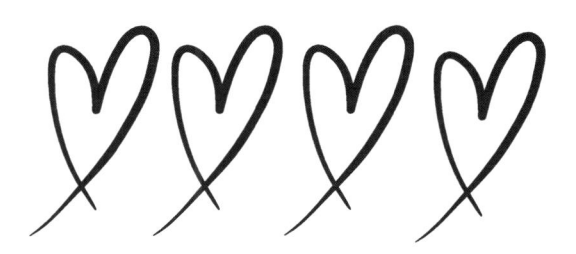

The Art of Becoming

DAY 97

DAILY CHECK IN: ✓

- WOKE UP EARLY
- WENT TO THE GYM
- MORNING ROUTINE
- NIGHT ROUTINE
- ATE HEALTHY WHOLE FOODS
- READ AT LEAST 10 PAGES OF ANY BOOK

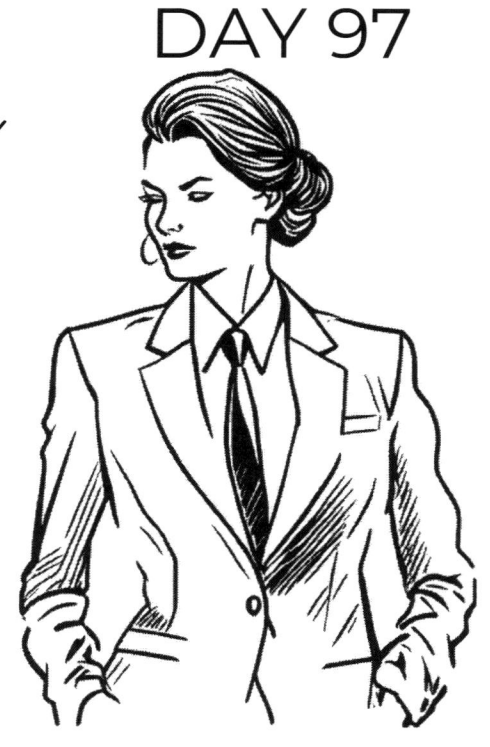

REFLECTIION:

_____
_____
_____
_____
_____
_____
_____
_____

TODAY'S AFFIRMATION

I CREATE SPACE FOR RELATIONSHIPS THAT BRING JOY INTO MY LIFE

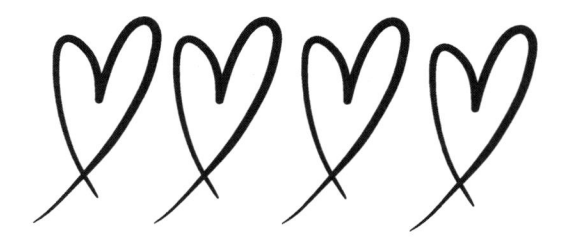

The Art of Becoming

DAY 98

DAILY CHECK IN: ✓

- WOKE UP EARLY
- WENT TO THE GYM
- MORNING ROUTINE
- NIGHT ROUTINE
- ATE HEALTHY WHOLE FOODS
- READ AT LEAST 10 PAGES OF ANY BOOK

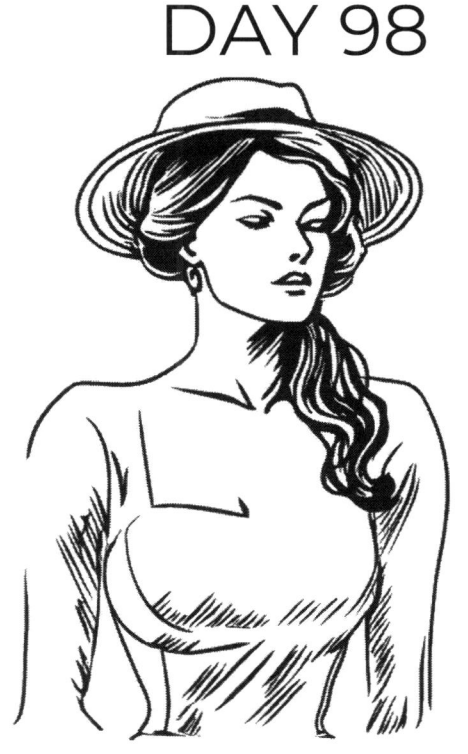

REFLECTIION:

_____
_____
_____
_____
_____
_____
_____
_____

TODAY'S AFFIRMATION

I
STAY
FOCUSED ON MY
GOALS
AND ELIMINATE
DISTRACTIONS

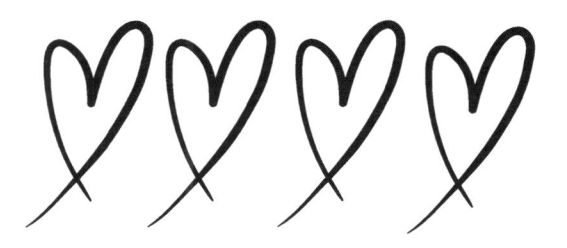

The Art of Becoming

DAY 99

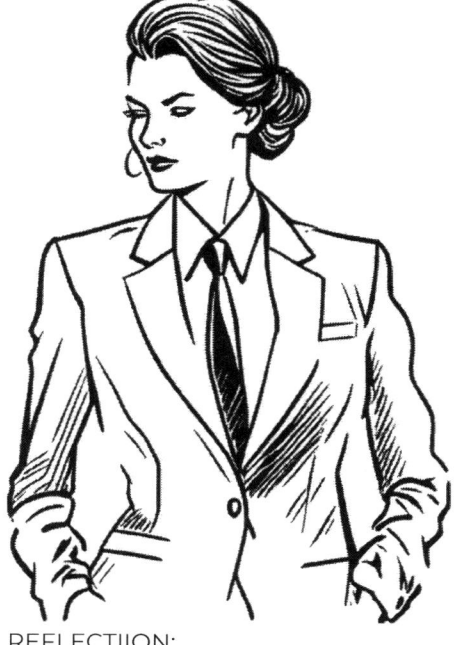

DAILY CHECK IN: ✓

- WOKE UP EARLY ☐
- WENT TO THE GYM ☐
- MORNING ROUTINE ☐
- NIGHT ROUTINE ☐
- ATE HEALTHY WHOLE FOODS ☐
- READ AT LEAST 10 PAGES OF ANY BOOK ☐

REFLECTIION:

_____
_____
_____
_____
_____
_____
_____
_____
_____
_____

TODAY'S AFFIRMATION

MY TIME IS VALUABLE, AND I USE IT WISELY

The Art of Becoming

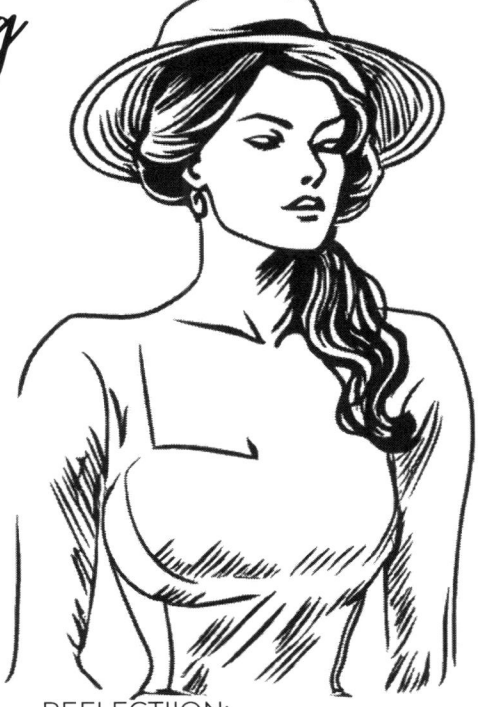

DAY 100

DAILY CHECK IN: ✓

- WOKE UP EARLY
- WENT TO THE GYM
- MORNING ROUTINE
- NIGHT ROUTINE
- ATE HEALTHY WHOLE FOODS
- READ AT LEAST 10 PAGES OF ANY BOOK

REFLECTIION:

_____
_____
_____
_____
_____
_____
_____
_____
_____

TODAY'S AFFIRMATION

I BREAK MY GOALS INTO SMALL, MANAGEABLE STEPS AND TAKE ACTION

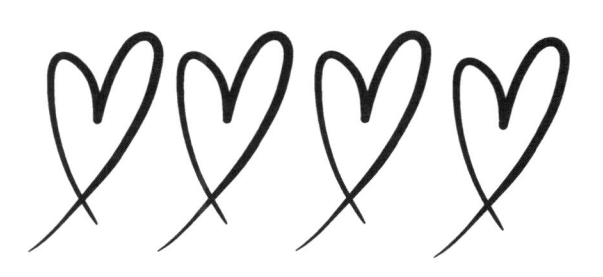

The Art of Becoming

DAY 101

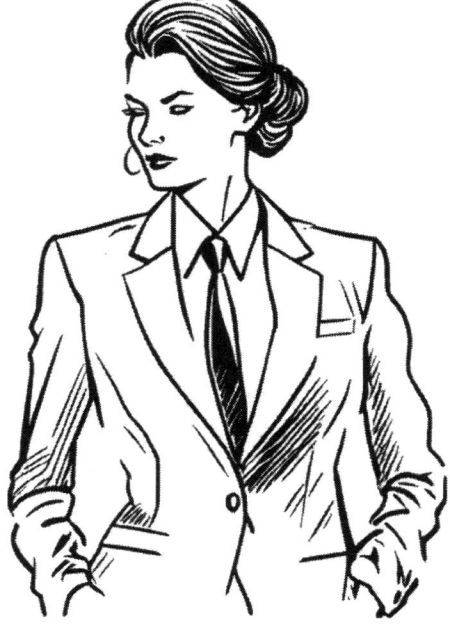

DAILY CHECK IN: ✓

- WOKE UP EARLY ☐
- WENT TO THE GYM ☐
- MORNING ROUTINE ☐
- NIGHT ROUTINE ☐
- ATE HEALTHY WHOLE FOODS ☐
- READ AT LEAST 10 PAGES OF ANY BOOK ☐

TODAY'S AFFIRMATION

I ATTRACT WEALTH AND ABUNDANCE EFFORTLESSLY

REFLECTIION:

_____
_____
_____
_____
_____
_____
_____
_____
_____

♡ ♡ ♡ ♡

The Art of Becoming

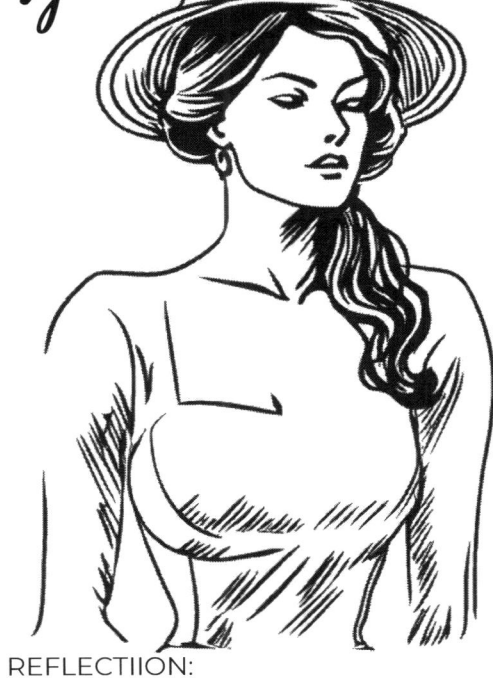

DAY 102

DAILY CHECK IN: ✓

- WOKE UP EARLY
- WENT TO THE GYM
- MORNING ROUTINE
- NIGHT ROUTINE
- ATE HEALTHY WHOLE FOODS
- READ AT LEAST 10 PAGES OF ANY BOOK

REFLECTIION:

_____
_____
_____
_____
_____
_____
_____
_____

TODAY'S AFFIRMATION

MONEY FLOWS TO ME IN EXPECTED AND UNEXPECTED WAYS

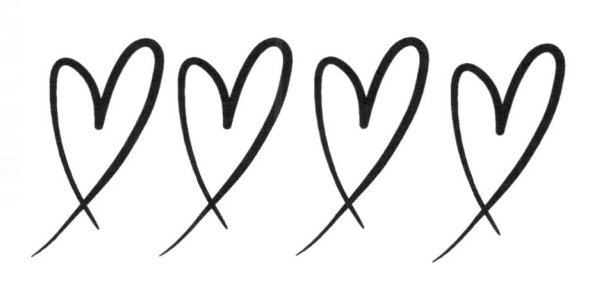

DAY 103

The Art of Becoming

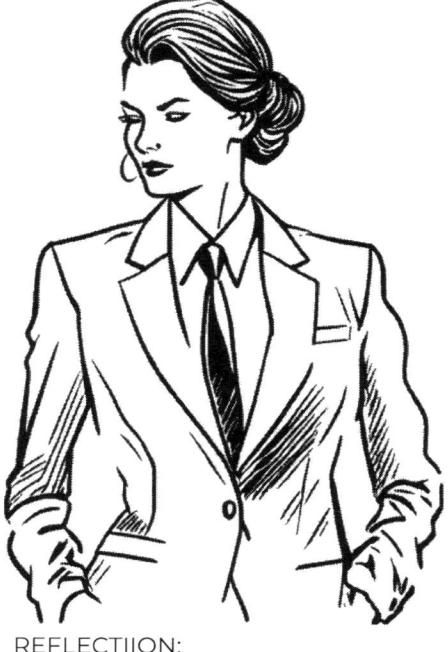

DAILY CHECK IN: ✓

- WOKE UP EARLY ☐
- WENT TO THE GYM ☐
- MORNING ROUTINE ☐
- NIGHT ROUTINE ☐
- ATE HEALTHY WHOLE FOODS ☐
- READ AT LEAST 10 PAGES OF ANY BOOK ☐

REFLECTIION: _____
_____
_____
_____
_____
_____
_____
_____
_____
_____

TODAY'S AFFIRMATION

I AM WORTHY OF FINANCIAL FREEDOM AND SUCCESS

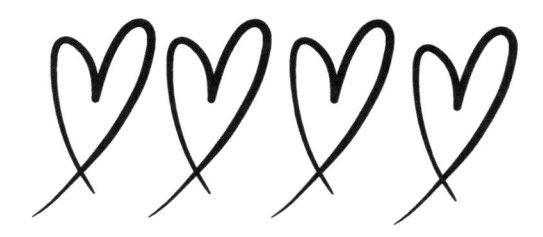

The Art of Becoming

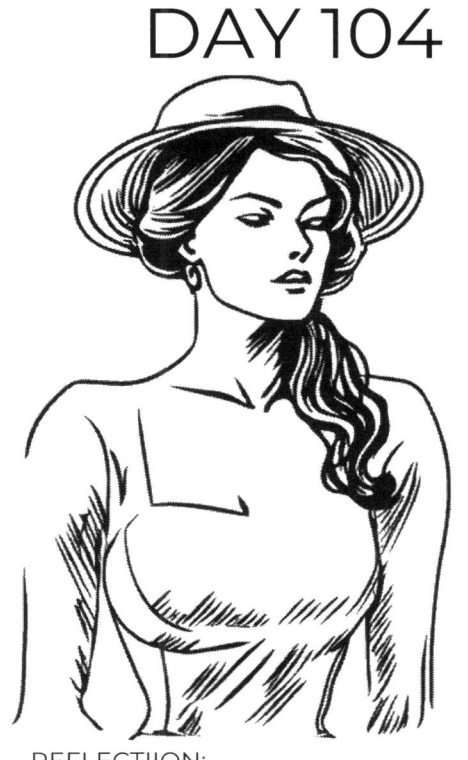

DAY 104

DAILY CHECK IN: ✓

- WOKE UP EARLY ☐
- WENT TO THE GYM ☐
- MORNING ROUTINE ☐
- NIGHT ROUTINE ☐
- ATE HEALTHY WHOLE FOODS ☐
- READ AT LEAST 10 PAGES OF ANY BOOK ☐

REFLECTIION:

_____
_____
_____
_____
_____
_____
_____
_____
_____

TODAY'S AFFIRMATION

MY
DREAMS
ARE BECOMING
MY
REALITY

The Art of Becoming

DAY 105

DAILY CHECK IN: ✓

- WOKE UP EARLY
- WENT TO THE GYM
- MORNING ROUTINE
- NIGHT ROUTINE
- ATE HEALTHY WHOLE FOODS
- READ AT LEAST 10 PAGES OF ANY BOOK

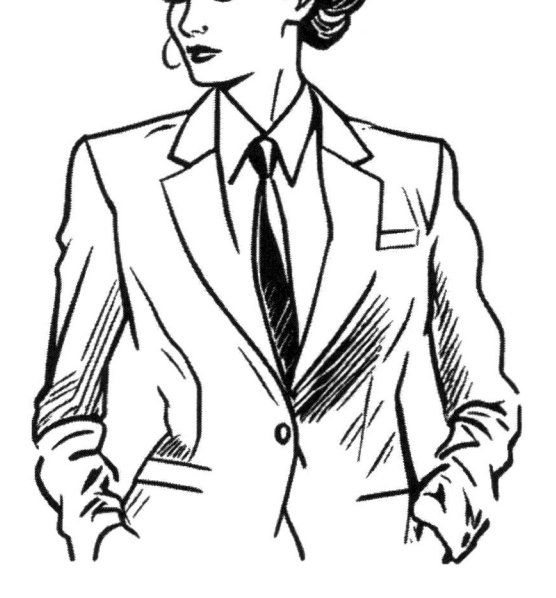

REFLECTIION:

TODAY'S AFFIRMATION

I AM STRONG, CAPABLE, AND RESILIENT

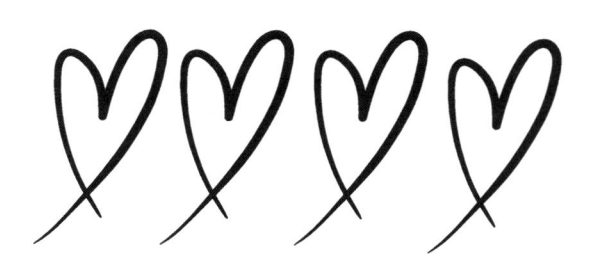

The Art of Becoming

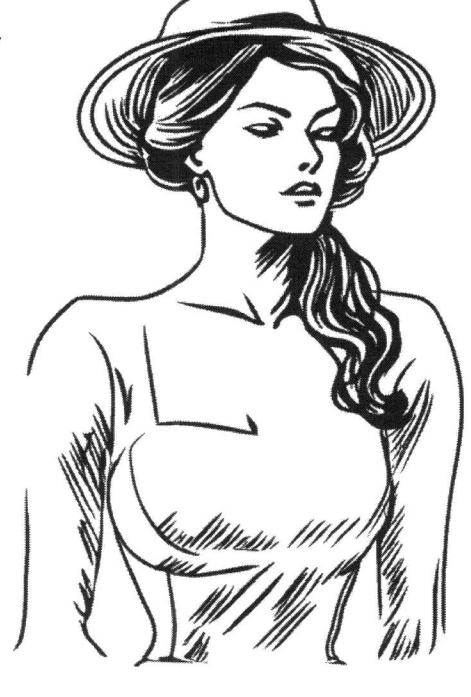

DAY 106

DAILY CHECK IN: ✓

- WOKE UP EARLY
- WENT TO THE GYM
- MORNING ROUTINE
- NIGHT ROUTINE
- ATE HEALTHY WHOLE FOODS
- READ AT LEAST 10 PAGES OF ANY BOOK

REFLECTIION:

_____
_____
_____
_____
_____
_____
_____
_____

TODAY'S AFFIRMATION

I
LET GO
OF WHAT I
CAN'T
CONTROL
AND TRUST THE
JOURNEY

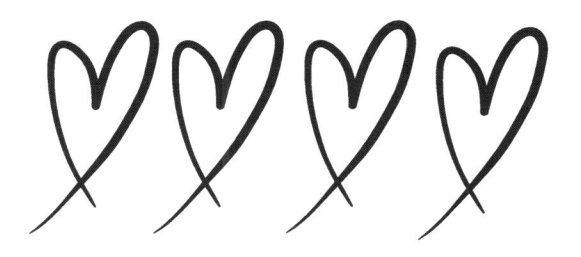

The Art of Becoming

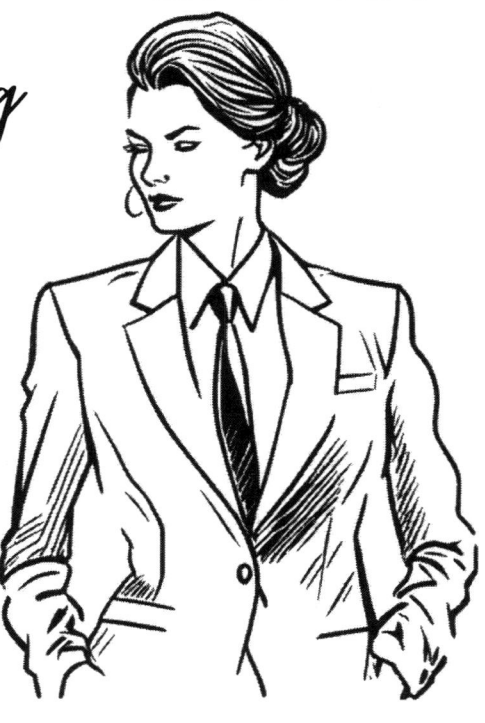

DAY 107

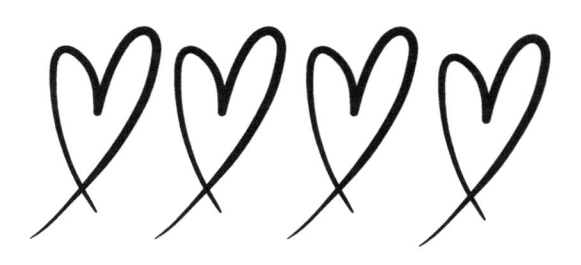

DAILY CHECK IN: ✓

- WOKE UP EARLY
- WENT TO THE GYM
- MORNING ROUTINE
- NIGHT ROUTINE
- ATE HEALTHY WHOLE FOODS
- READ AT LEAST 10 PAGES OF ANY BOOK

REFLECTIION:

_____
_____
_____
_____
_____
_____
_____
_____
_____
_____

TODAY'S AFFIRMATION

I AM GRATEFUL FOR EVERYTHING I HAVE AND EVERYTHING I'M BECOMING

The Art of Becoming

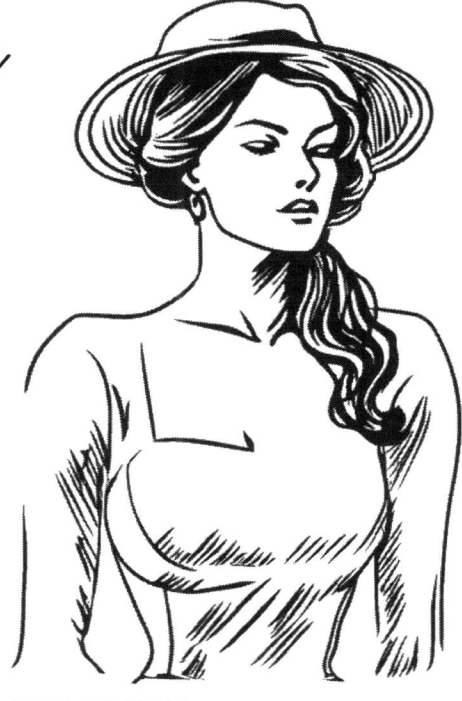

DAY 108

DAILY CHECK IN: ✓

- WOKE UP EARLY
- WENT TO THE GYM
- MORNING ROUTINE
- NIGHT ROUTINE
- ATE HEALTHY WHOLE FOODS
- READ AT LEAST 10 PAGES OF ANY BOOK

REFLECTIION:

_____
_____
_____
_____
_____
_____
_____
_____
_____

TODAY'S AFFIRMATION

I
CHOOSE
JOY
IN EVERY MOMENT

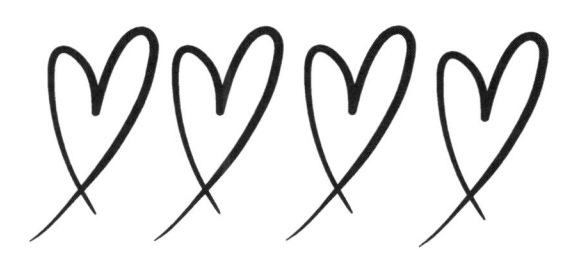

DAY 109

The Art of Becoming

DAILY CHECK IN: ✓

- WOKE UP EARLY ☐
- WENT TO THE GYM ☐
- MORNING ROUTINE ☐
- NIGHT ROUTINE ☐
- ATE HEALTHY WHOLE FOODS ☐
- READ AT LEAST 10 PAGES OF ANY BOOK ☐

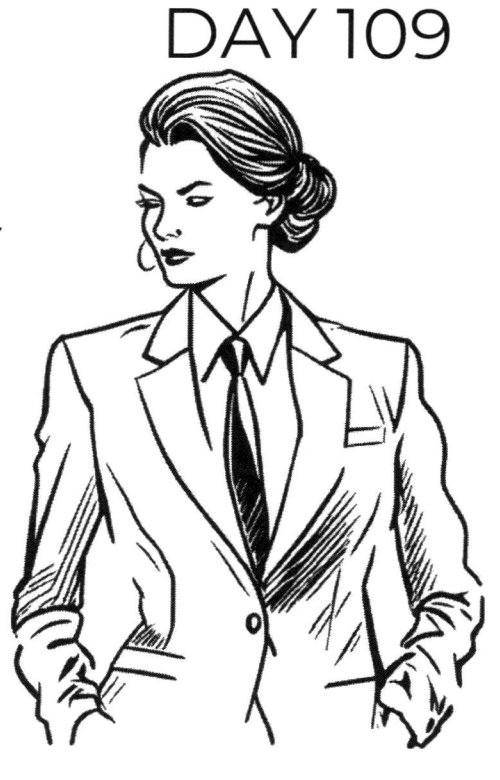

REFLECTIION:
_____
_____
_____
_____
_____
_____
_____
_____
_____
_____

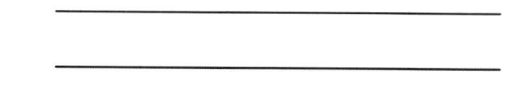

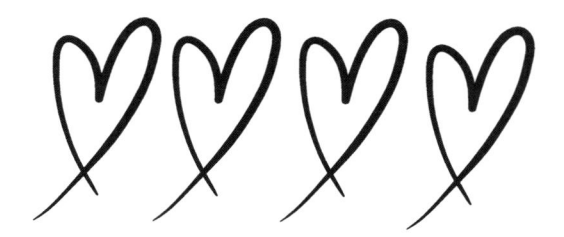

TODAY'S AFFIRMATION

I APPRECIATE THE LITTLE THINGS THAT MAKE LIFE BEAUTIFUL

The Art of Becoming

DAY 110

DAILY CHECK IN: ✓

- WOKE UP EARLY
- WENT TO THE GYM
- MORNING ROUTINE
- NIGHT ROUTINE
- ATE HEALTHY WHOLE FOODS
- READ AT LEAST 10 PAGES OF ANY BOOK

REFLECTIION:
_____
_____
_____
_____
_____
_____
_____
_____

TODAY'S AFFIRMATION

I
COMMIT
TO THE PROCESS
AND
TRUST MYSELF

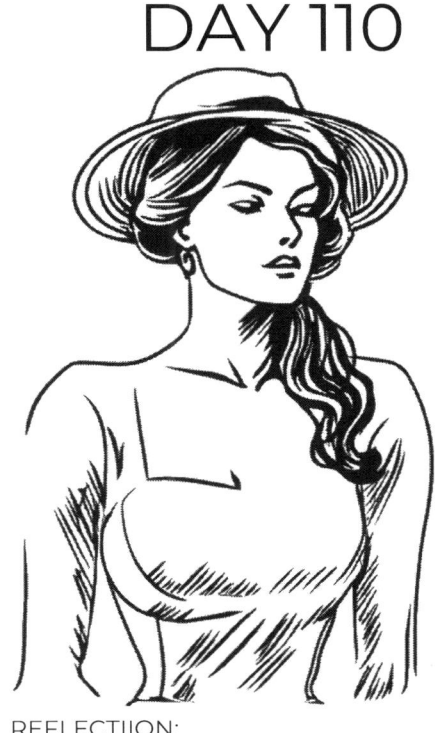

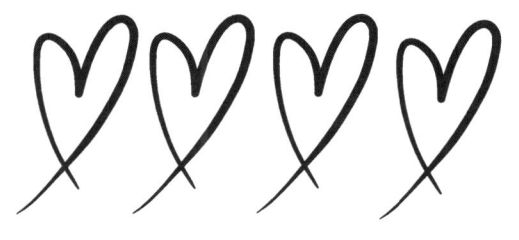

The Art of Becoming

DAY 111

DAILY CHECK IN: ✓

- WOKE UP EARLY ☐
- WENT TO THE GYM ☐
- MORNING ROUTINE ☐
- NIGHT ROUTINE ☐
- ATE HEALTHY WHOLE FOODS ☐
- READ AT LEAST 10 PAGES OF ANY BOOK ☐

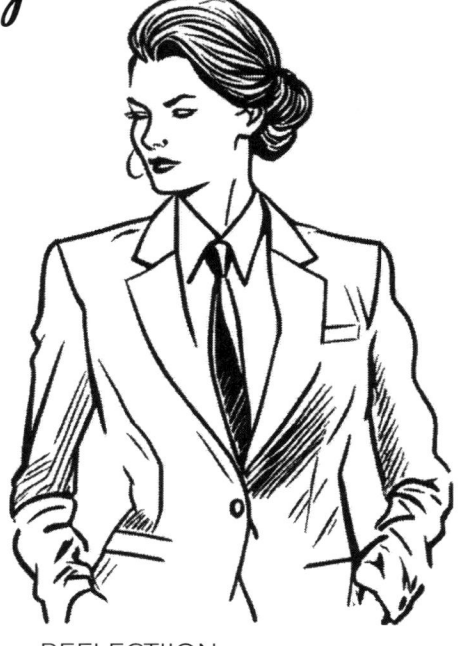

REFLECTIION:

_____
_____
_____
_____
_____
_____
_____
_____
_____

TODAY'S AFFIRMATION

I AM STEPPING INTO THE HIGHEST VERSION OF MYSELF EVERY DAY

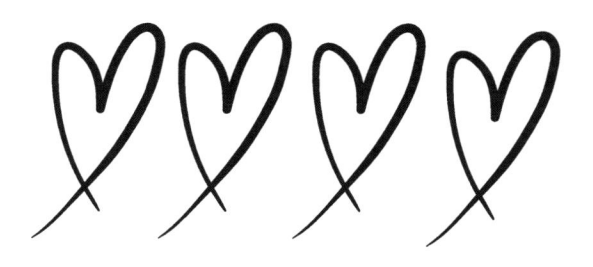

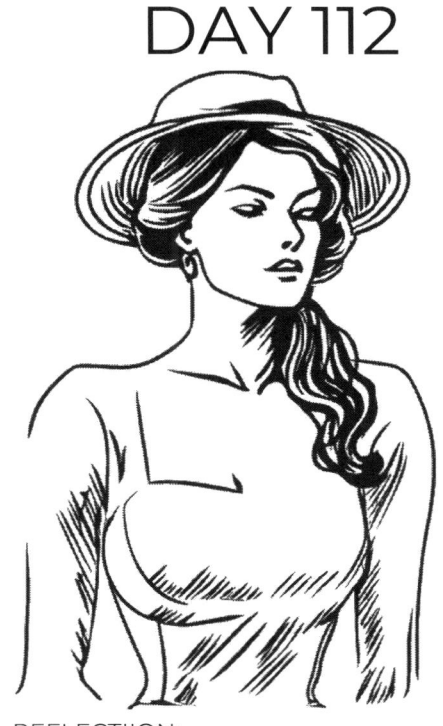

The Art of Becoming

DAY 112

DAILY CHECK IN: ✓
___

- WOKE UP EARLY

- WENT TO THE GYM

- MORNING ROUTINE

- NIGHT ROUTINE

- ATE HEALTHY WHOLE FOODS

- READ AT LEAST 10 PAGES OF ANY BOOK

REFLECTIION:
___
___
___
___
___
___
___
___
___

TODAY'S AFFIRMATION
___

I
AM
OPEN TO
RECEIVING
UNLIMITED
ABUNDANCE

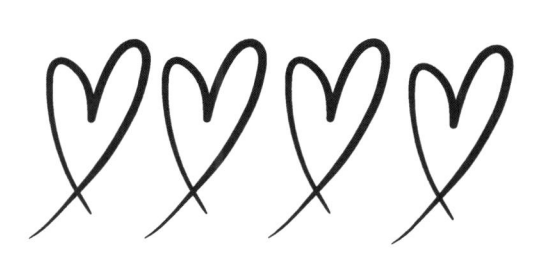

The Art of Becoming

DAY 113

DAILY CHECK IN: ✓

- WOKE UP EARLY
- WENT TO THE GYM
- MORNING ROUTINE
- NIGHT ROUTINE
- ATE HEALTHY WHOLE FOODS
- READ AT LEAST 10 PAGES OF ANY BOOK

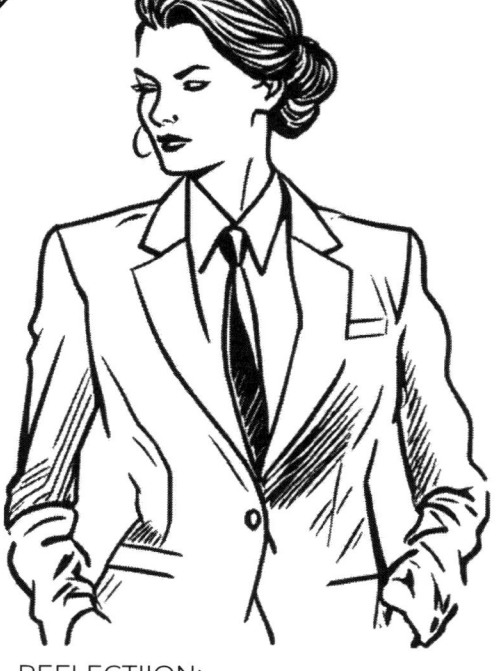

REFLECTIION:

_____
_____
_____
_____
_____
_____
_____
_____

TODAY'S AFFIRMATION

I MANIFEST MY DREAM LIFE THROUGH BELIEF AND ACTION

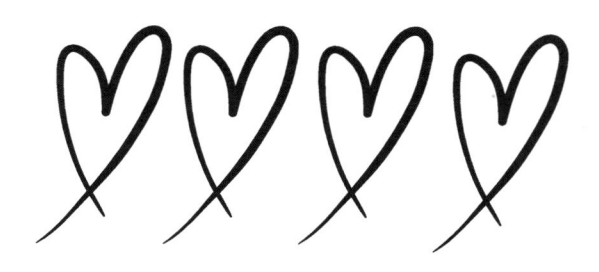

The Art of Becoming

DAY 114

DAILY CHECK IN: ✓

- WOKE UP EARLY
- WENT TO THE GYM
- MORNING ROUTINE
- NIGHT ROUTINE
- ATE HEALTHY WHOLE FOODS
- READ AT LEAST 10 PAGES OF ANY BOOK

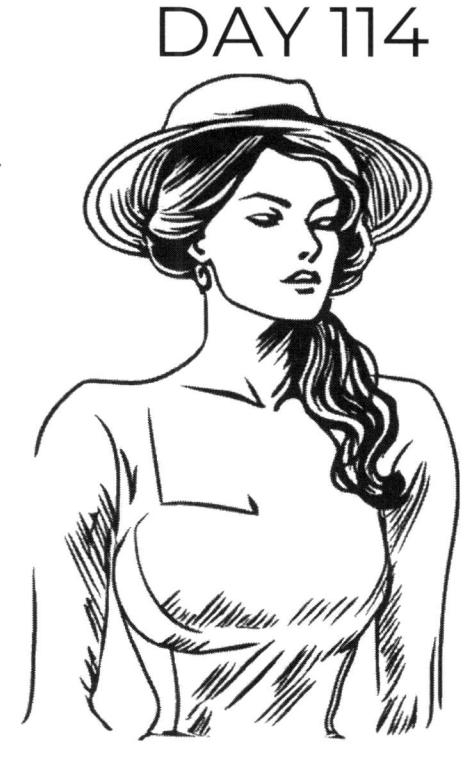

REFLECTIION:

_____
_____
_____
_____
_____
_____
_____
_____
_____
_____

TODAY'S AFFIRMATION

I TRUST THAT EVERYTHING I DESIRE IS MAKING IT'S WAY TO ME

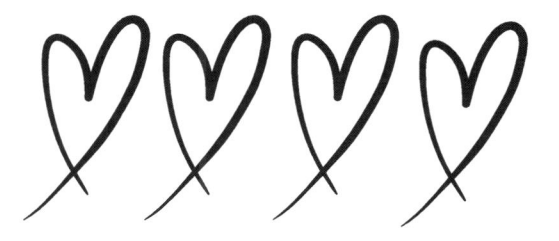

The Art of Becoming

DAY 115

DAILY CHECK IN: ✓

- WOKE UP EARLY ☐
- WENT TO THE GYM ☐
- MORNING ROUTINE ☐
- NIGHT ROUTINE ☐
- ATE HEALTHY WHOLE FOODS ☐
- READ AT LEAST 10 PAGES OF ANY BOOK ☐

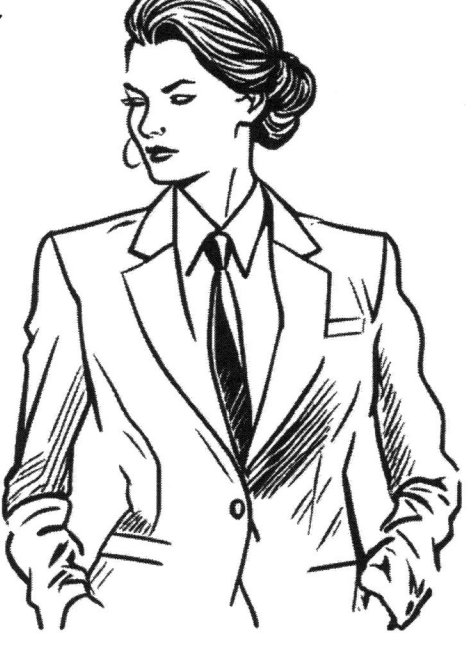

REFLECTIION:

_____
_____
_____
_____
_____
_____
_____
_____
_____

TODAY'S AFFIRMATION

I
ALIGN MY
THOUGHTS AND
ACTIONS
WITH
THE LIFE I DESIRE

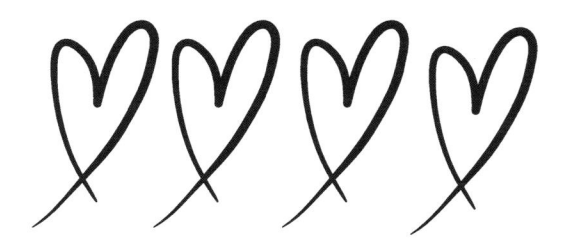

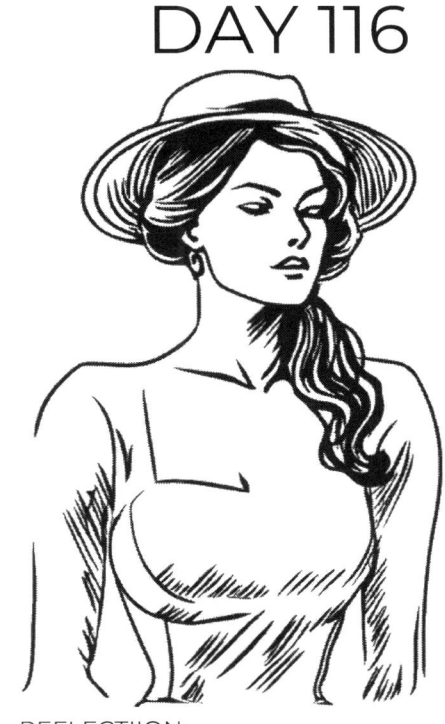

The Art of Becoming

DAY 116

DAILY CHECK IN: ✓

- WOKE UP EARLY
- WENT TO THE GYM
- MORNING ROUTINE
- NIGHT ROUTINE
- ATE HEALTHY WHOLE FOODS
- READ AT LEAST 10 PAGES OF ANY BOOK

REFLECTIION:

_____
_____
_____
_____
_____
_____
_____
_____
_____

TODAY'S AFFIRMATION

I ATTRACT OPPORTUNITIES THAT ALIGN WITH MY HIGHEST GOOD

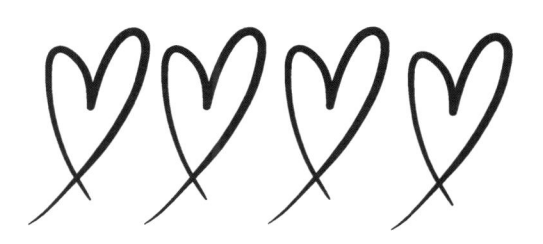

DAY 117

The Art of Becoming

DAILY CHECK IN: ✓

- WOKE UP EARLY
- WENT TO THE GYM
- MORNING ROUTINE
- NIGHT ROUTINE
- ATE HEALTHY WHOLE FOODS
- READ AT LEAST 10 PAGES OF ANY BOOK

REFLECTIION:

_____
_____
_____
_____
_____
_____
_____
_____
_____
_____

TODAY'S AFFIRMATION

I DESERVE TO LIVE A LIFE OF FINANCIAL FREEDOM AND EASE

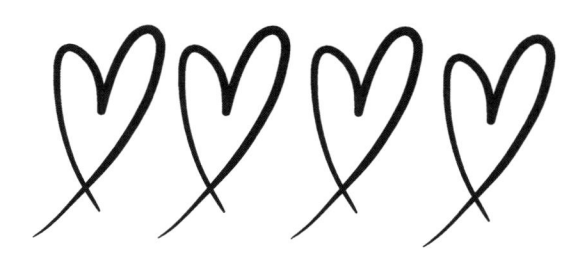

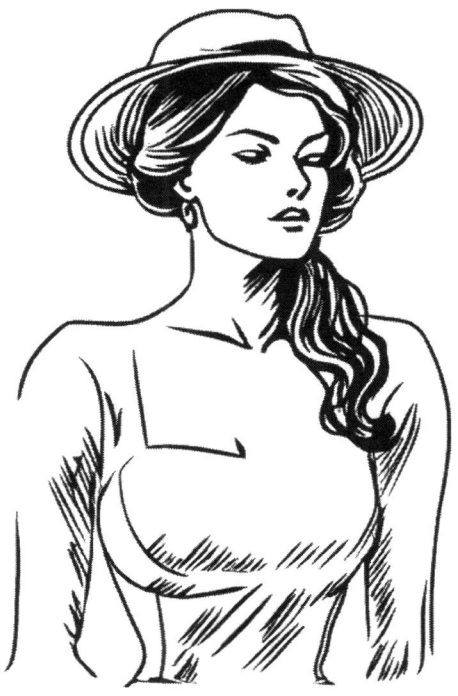

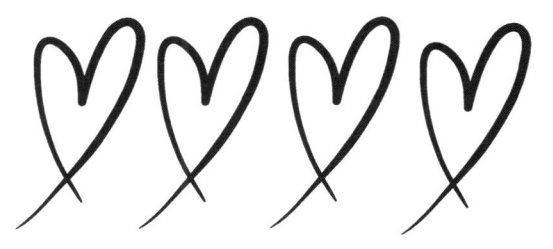

The Art of Becoming

DAY 118

DAILY CHECK IN: ✓

- WOKE UP EARLY
- WENT TO THE GYM
- MORNING ROUTINE
- NIGHT ROUTINE
- ATE HEALTHY WHOLE FOODS
- READ AT LEAST 10 PAGES OF ANY BOOK

REFLECTIION:

_____
_____
_____
_____
_____
_____
_____
_____

TODAY'S AFFIRMATION

I
AM A
MAGNET FOR
PROSPERITY
AND
JOY

The Art of Becoming

DAY 119

DAILY CHECK IN: ✓

- WOKE UP EARLY
- WENT TO THE GYM
- MORNING ROUTINE
- NIGHT ROUTINE
- ATE HEALTHY WHOLE FOODS
- READ AT LEAST 10 PAGES OF ANY BOOK

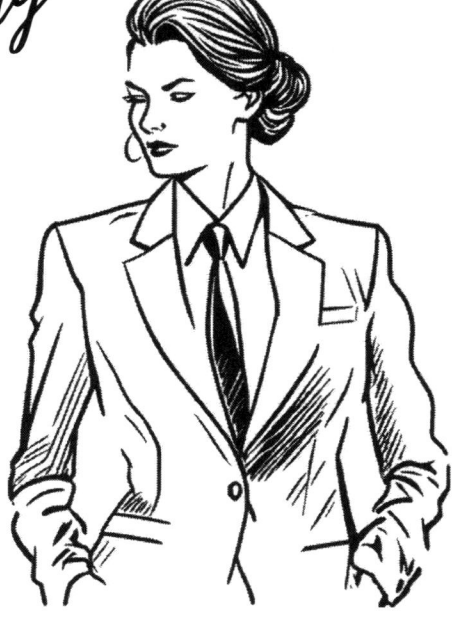

REFLECTIION:
_____
_____
_____
_____
_____
_____
_____
_____
_____

TODAY'S AFFIRMATION

I AM IN ALIGNMENT WITH THE FREQUENCY OF WEALTH

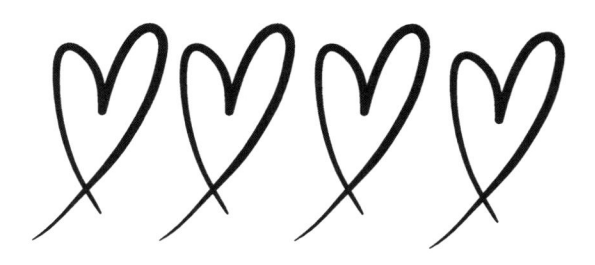

DAY 120

The Art of Becoming

DAILY CHECK IN: ✓

- WOKE UP EARLY
- WENT TO THE GYM
- MORNING ROUTINE
- NIGHT ROUTINE
- ATE HEALTHY WHOLE FOODS
- READ AT LEAST 10 PAGES OF ANY BOOK

MAINTENANCE DAY TIME TO VISIT THE BEAUTY PARLOR, BABES!

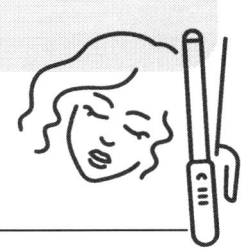

REFLECTIION:

_____
_____
_____

_____
_____
_____
_____
_____

TODAY'S AFFIRMATION

I BREAK MY GOALS INTO SMALL, MANAGEABLE STEPS AND TAKE ACTION

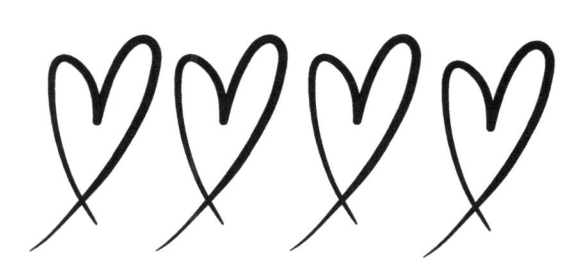

The Art of Becoming

DAY 121

DAILY CHECK IN: ✓

- WOKE UP EARLY
- WENT TO THE GYM
- MORNING ROUTINE
- NIGHT ROUTINE
- ATE HEALTHY WHOLE FOODS
- READ AT LEAST 10 PAGES OF ANY BOOK

REFLECTIION:

_____
_____
_____
_____
_____
_____
_____
_____
_____

TODAY'S AFFIRMATION

I
RELEASE ALL FEAR
AND
TRUST
THAT I AM
SUPPORTED

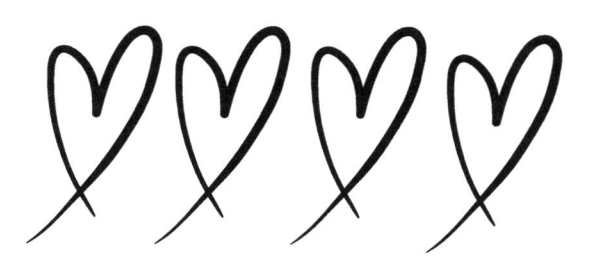

DAY 122

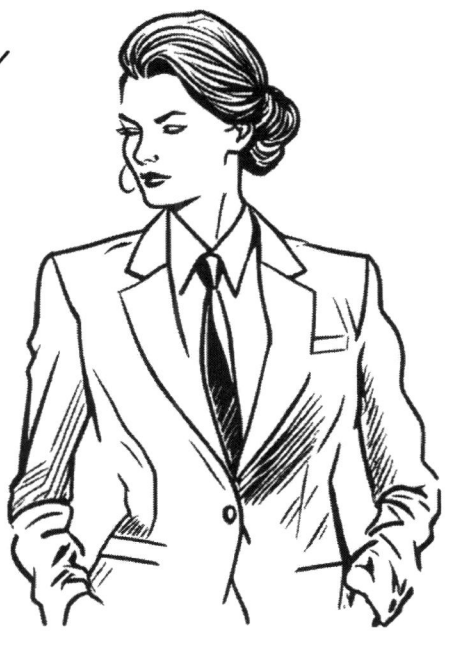

The Art of Becoming

DAILY CHECK IN: ✓

- WOKE UP EARLY
- WENT TO THE GYM
- MORNING ROUTINE
- NIGHT ROUTINE
- ATE HEALTHY WHOLE FOODS
- READ AT LEAST 10 PAGES OF ANY BOOK

REFLECTIION:

_____
_____
_____
_____
_____
_____
_____
_____

TODAY'S AFFIRMATION

MY SETBACKS ARE SETUPS FOR GREATER COMEBACKS

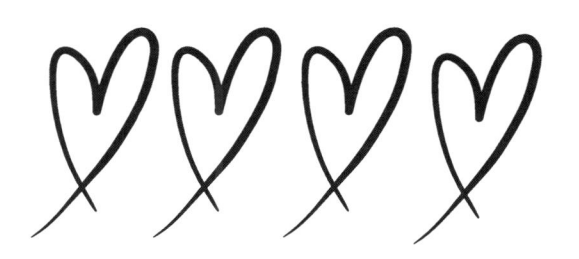

DAY 123

The Art of Becoming

DAILY CHECK IN: ✓

- WOKE UP EARLY
- WENT TO THE GYM
- MORNING ROUTINE
- NIGHT ROUTINE
- ATE HEALTHY WHOLE FOODS
- READ AT LEAST 10 PAGES OF ANY BOOK

REFLECTIION:

_____
_____
_____
_____
_____
_____
_____
_____
_____

TODAY'S AFFIRMATION

I EMBRACE DISCOMFORT BECAUSE IT LEADS TO MY EXPANSION

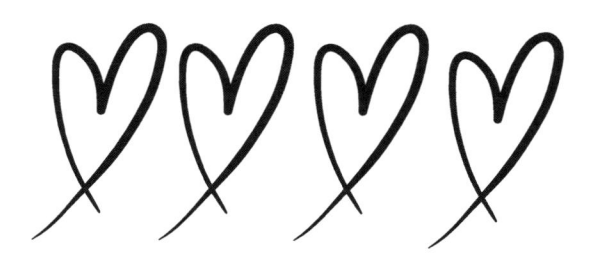

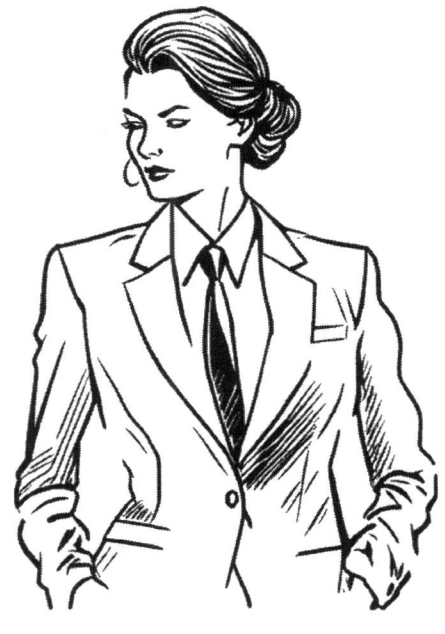

The Art of Becoming

DAY 124

DAILY CHECK IN: ✓
_____

- WOKE UP EARLY

- WENT TO THE GYM

- MORNING ROUTINE

- NIGHT ROUTINE

- ATE HEALTHY WHOLE FOODS

- READ AT LEAST 10 PAGES OF ANY BOOK

REFLECTIION:
_____
_____
_____
_____
_____
_____
_____
_____

TODAY'S AFFIRMATION
_____

I
AM AT PEACE
WITH WHERE I AM
WHILE
STRIVING FOR WHERE
I
WANT TO BE

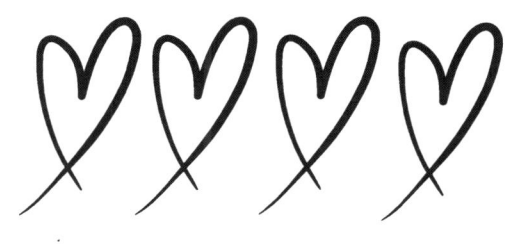

The Art of Becoming

DAY 125

DAILY CHECK IN: ✓

- WOKE UP EARLY
- WENT TO THE GYM
- MORNING ROUTINE
- NIGHT ROUTINE
- ATE HEALTHY WHOLE FOODS
- READ AT LEAST 10 PAGES OF ANY BOOK

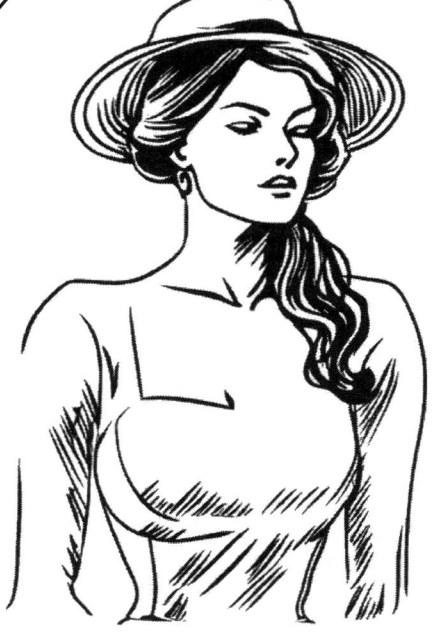

REFLECTIION:
_____
_____
_____
_____
_____
_____
_____
_____
_____
_____

TODAY'S AFFIRMATION

MY STRENGTH IS GREATER THAN ANY CHALLENGE I FACE

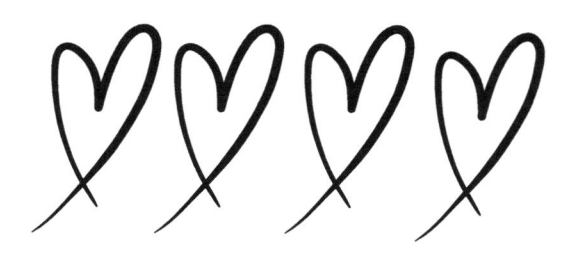

The Art of Becoming

DAY 126

DAILY CHECK IN: ✓

- WOKE UP EARLY
- WENT TO THE GYM
- MORNING ROUTINE
- NIGHT ROUTINE
- ATE HEALTHY WHOLE FOODS
- READ AT LEAST 10 PAGES OF ANY BOOK

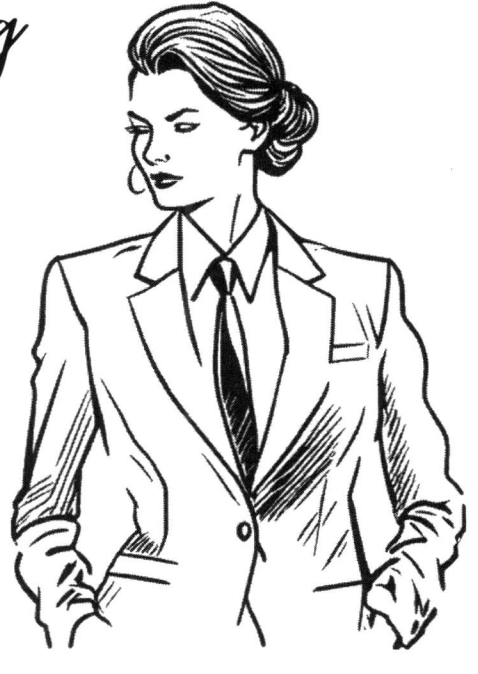

REFLECTIION:

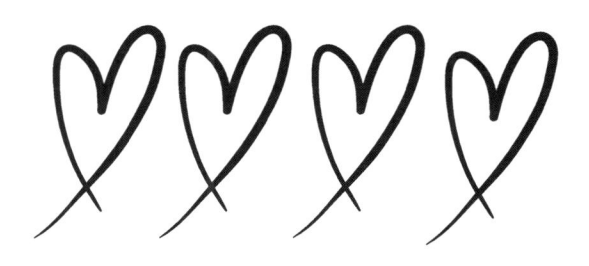

_____
_____
_____
_____
_____
_____
_____
_____
_____

TODAY'S AFFIRMATION

I LEARN AND GROW FROM ANY EXPERIENCE, GOOD OR BAD

The Art of Becoming

DAY 127

DAILY CHECK IN: ✓

- WOKE UP EARLY
- WENT TO THE GYM
- MORNING ROUTINE
- NIGHT ROUTINE
- ATE HEALTHY WHOLE FOODS
- READ AT LEAST 10 PAGES OF ANY BOOK

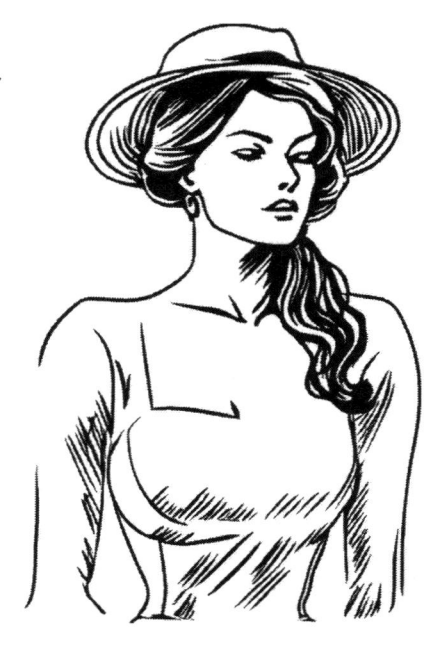

REFLECTIION:

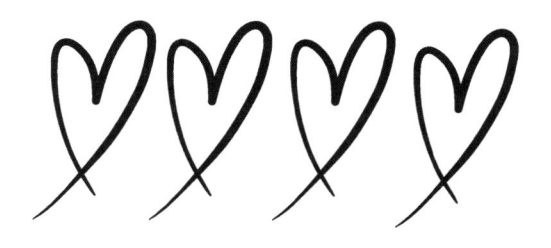

_____
_____
_____
_____
_____
_____
_____
_____

TODAY'S AFFIRMATION

I DO NOT LET REJECTION SHAKE MY CONFIDENCE - IT ONLY REDIRECTS ME

The Art of Becoming

DAY 128

DAILY CHECK IN: ✓

- WOKE UP EARLY
- WENT TO THE GYM
- MORNING ROUTINE
- NIGHT ROUTINE
- ATE HEALTHY WHOLE FOODS
- READ AT LEAST 10 PAGES OF ANY BOOK

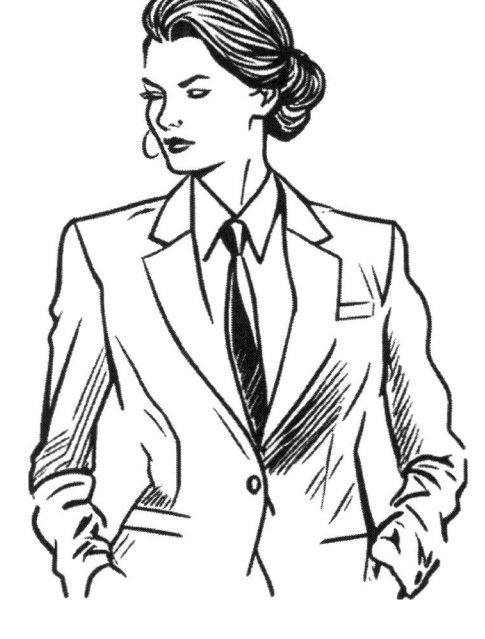

REFLECTIION:
_____
_____
_____
_____
_____
_____
_____
_____
_____

TODAY'S AFFIRMATION

I ALLOW MYSELF TO FEEL, HEAL, AND MOVE FOWARD

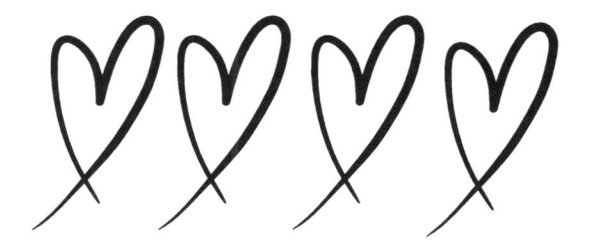

The Art of Becoming

DAY 129

DAILY CHECK IN: ✓

- WOKE UP EARLY ☐
- WENT TO THE GYM ☐
- MORNING ROUTINE ☐
- NIGHT ROUTINE ☐
- ATE HEALTHY WHOLE FOODS ☐
- READ AT LEAST 10 PAGES OF ANY BOOK ☐

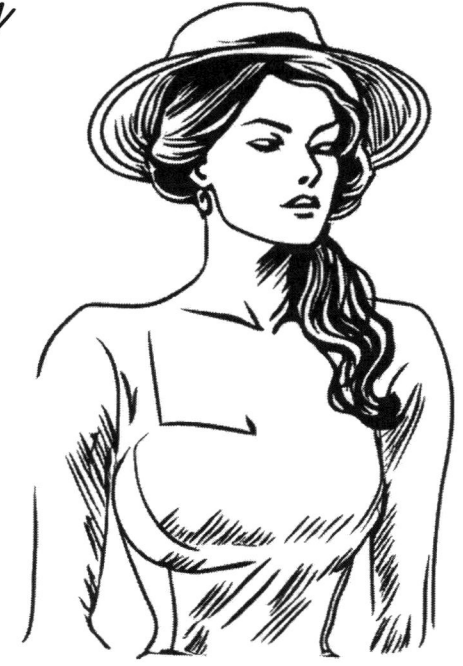

REFLECTIION:

_____
_____
_____
_____
_____
_____
_____
_____
_____

TODAY'S AFFIRMATION

I FIND BEAUTY IN THE PRESENT MOMENT

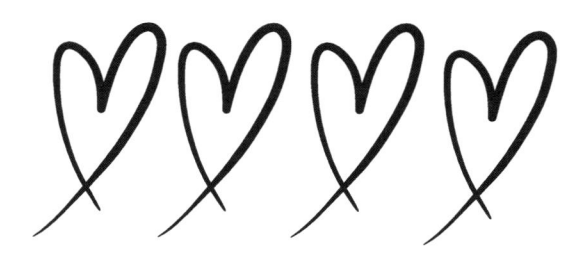

♡ ♡ ♡ ♡

The Art of Becoming

DAY 130

DAILY CHECK IN: ✓

- WOKE UP EARLY
- WENT TO THE GYM
- MORNING ROUTINE
- NIGHT ROUTINE
- ATE HEALTHY WHOLE FOODS
- READ AT LEAST 10 PAGES OF ANY BOOK

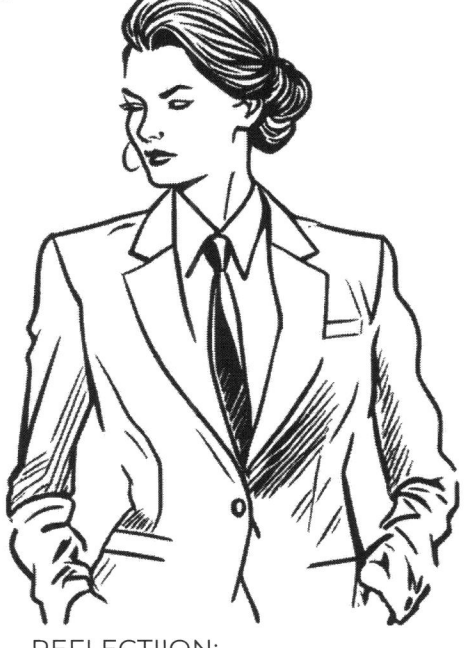

REFLECTIION:

_____
_____
_____
_____
_____
_____
_____
_____

TODAY'S AFFIRMATION

I APPRECIATE THE JOURNEY AS MUCH AS THE DESTINATION

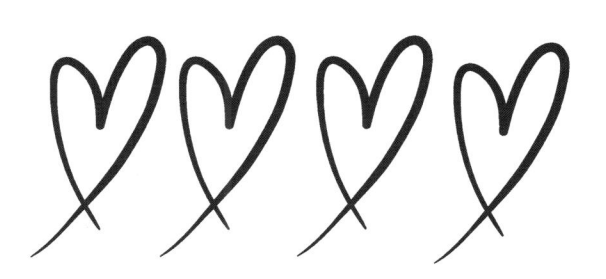

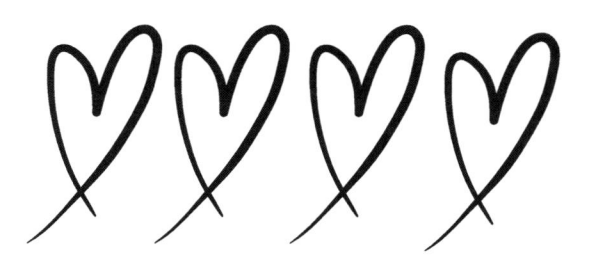

The Art of Becoming

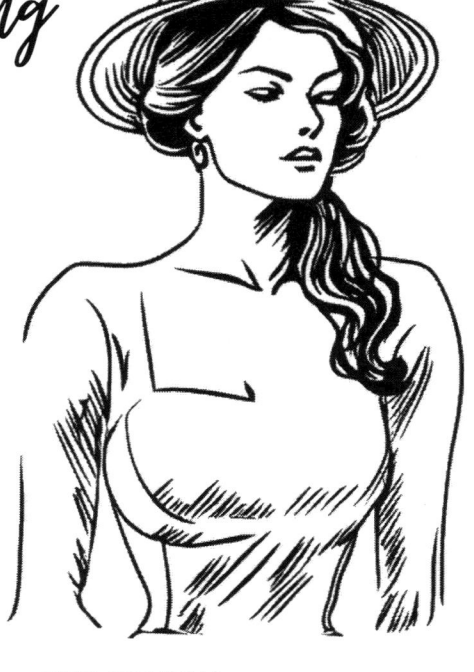

DAY 131

DAILY CHECK IN: ✓

- WOKE UP EARLY ☐
- WENT TO THE GYM ☐
- MORNING ROUTINE ☐
- NIGHT ROUTINE ☐
- ATE HEALTHY WHOLE FOODS ☐
- READ AT LEAST 10 PAGES OF ANY BOOK ☐

REFLECTIION:

_____
_____
_____
_____
_____
_____
_____
_____
_____

TODAY'S AFFIRMATION

MY
HEART IS FULL OF
GRATITUDE
FOR THE LIFE
I
AM CREATING

The Art of Becoming

DAY 132

DAILY CHECK IN: ✓

- WOKE UP EARLY
- WENT TO THE GYM
- MORNING ROUTINE
- NIGHT ROUTINE
- ATE HEALTHY WHOLE FOODS
- READ AT LEAST 10 PAGES OF ANY BOOK

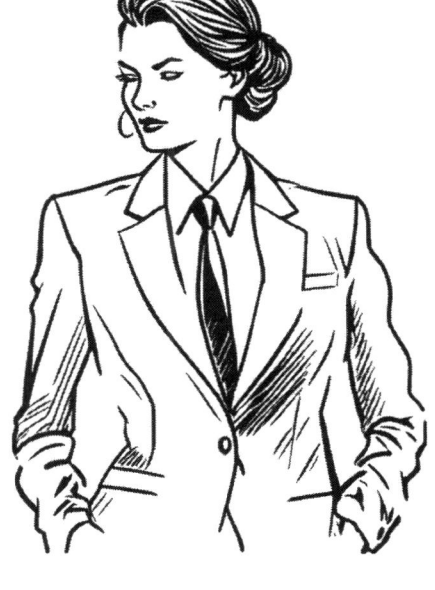

REFLECTIION:

_____
_____
_____
_____
_____
_____
_____
_____
_____

TODAY'S AFFIRMATION

I
FOCUS
ON THE GOOD
IN
EVERY SITUATION

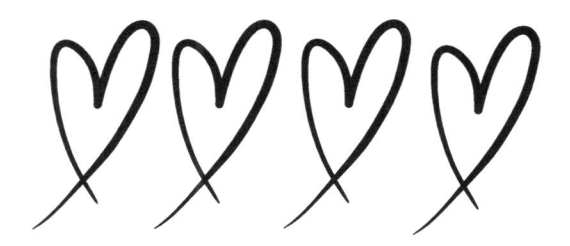

DAY 133

The Art of Becoming

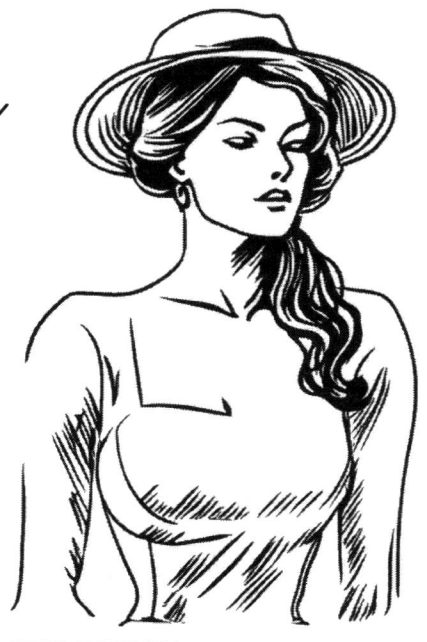

DAILY CHECK IN: ✓

- WOKE UP EARLY ☐
- WENT TO THE GYM ☐
- MORNING ROUTINE ☐
- NIGHT ROUTINE ☐
- ATE HEALTHY WHOLE FOODS ☐
- READ AT LEAST 10 PAGES OF ANY BOOK ☐

REFLECTIION:
_____
_____
_____
_____
_____
_____
_____
_____
_____

TODAY'S AFFIRMATION

I AM GRATEFUL FOR THE LOVE, SUPPORT, AND BLESSINGS IN MY LIFE

The Art of Becoming

DAY 134

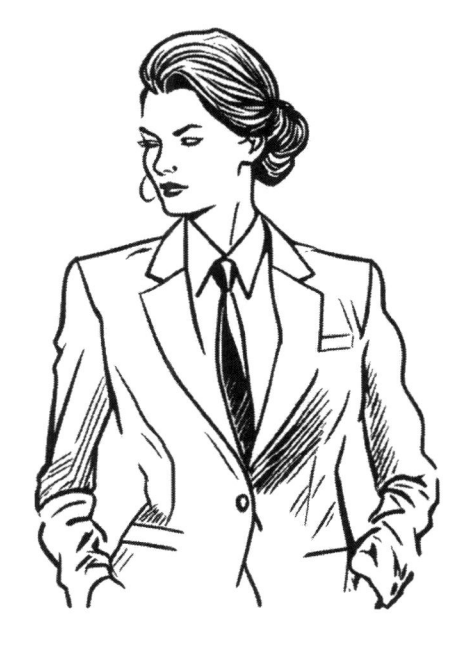

DAILY CHECK IN: ✓

- WOKE UP EARLY
- WENT TO THE GYM
- MORNING ROUTINE
- NIGHT ROUTINE
- ATE HEALTHY WHOLE FOODS
- READ AT LEAST 10 PAGES OF ANY BOOK

REFLECTIION:

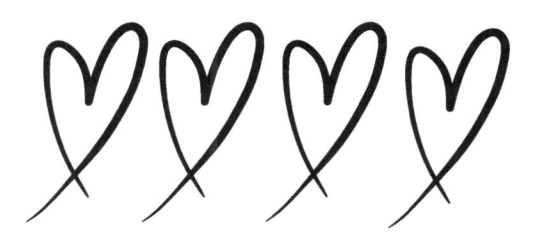

_____
_____
_____
_____
_____
_____
_____
_____
_____

TODAY'S AFFIRMATION

HAPPINESS
IS A CHOICE
AND
I CHOOSE IT
DAILY

DAY 135

The Art of Becoming

DAILY CHECK IN: ✓

- WOKE UP EARLY
- WENT TO THE GYM
- MORNING ROUTINE
- NIGHT ROUTINE
- ATE HEALTHY WHOLE FOODS
- READ AT LEAST 10 PAGES OF ANY BOOK

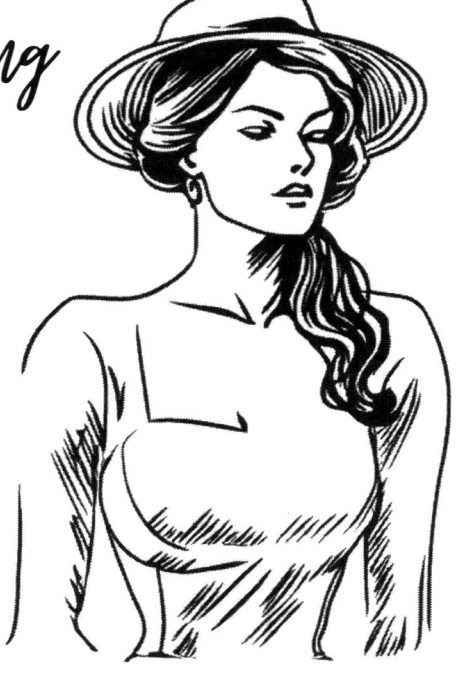

REFLECTIION:

_____
_____
_____
_____
_____
_____
_____
_____
_____

TODAY'S AFFIRMATION

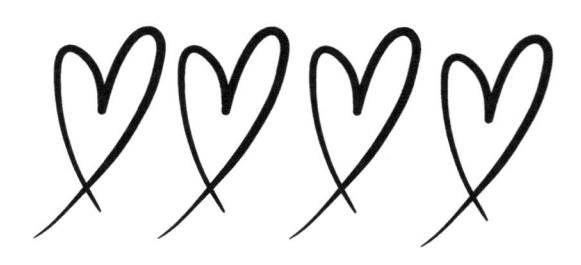

THE MORE I APPRECIATE LIFE, THE MORE IT GIVES ME TO CELEBRATE

The Art of Becoming

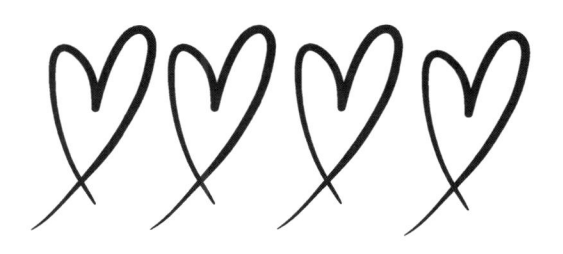

DAY 136

DAILY CHECK IN: ✓

- WOKE UP EARLY
- WENT TO THE GYM
- MORNING ROUTINE
- NIGHT ROUTINE
- ATE HEALTHY WHOLE FOODS
- READ AT LEAST 10 PAGES OF ANY BOOK

REFLECTIION:
_____
_____
_____
_____
_____
_____
_____
_____
_____

TODAY'S AFFIRMATION

I AM GRATEFUL FOR MY GROWTH AND TRANSFORMATION

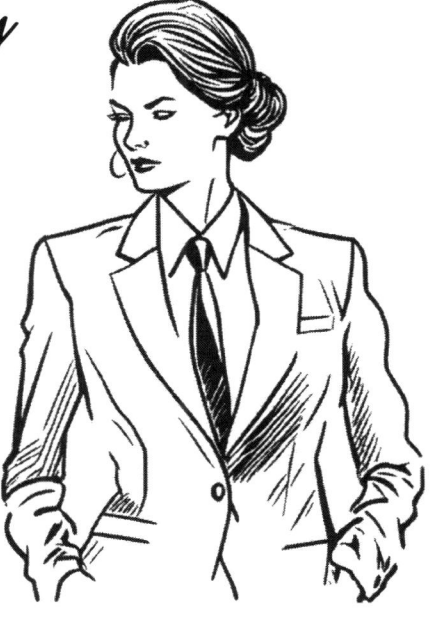

The Art of Becoming

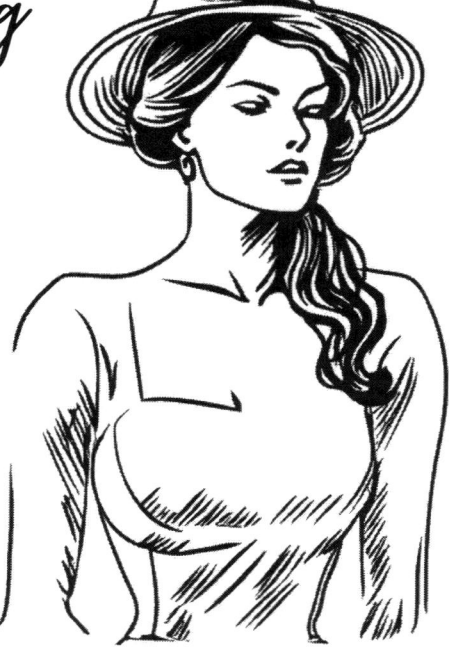

DAY 137

DAILY CHECK IN: ✓

- WOKE UP EARLY
- WENT TO THE GYM
- MORNING ROUTINE
- NIGHT ROUTINE
- ATE HEALTHY WHOLE FOODS
- READ AT LEAST 10 PAGES OF ANY BOOK

REFLECTIION:

_____
_____
_____
_____
_____
_____
_____
_____
_____
_____

TODAY'S AFFIRMATION

I FOCUS ON WHAT I HAVE, RATHER THAN WHAT I LACK

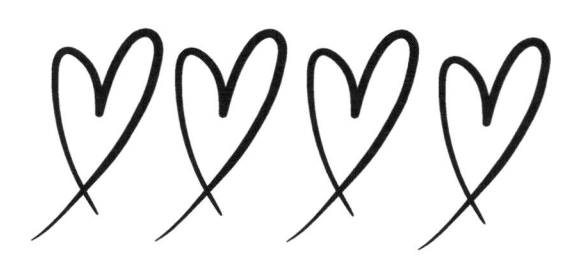

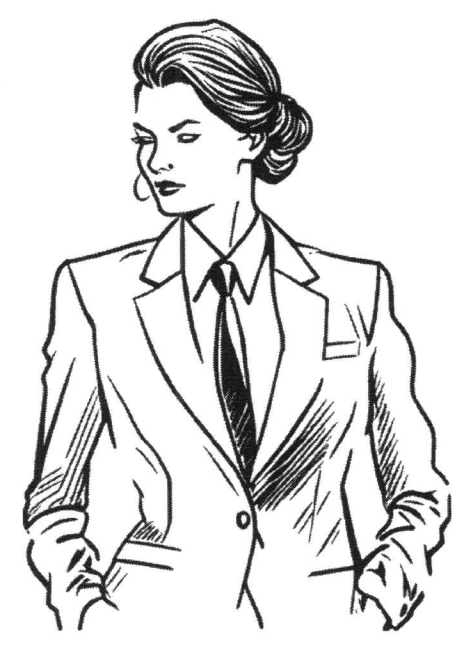

The Art of Becoming

DAY 138

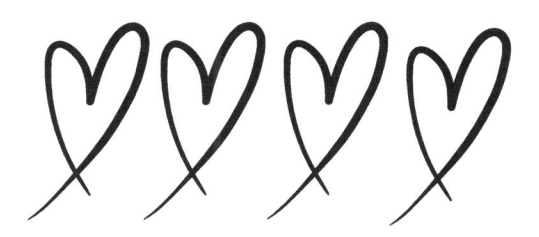

DAILY CHECK IN: ✓

- WOKE UP EARLY
- WENT TO THE GYM
- MORNING ROUTINE
- NIGHT ROUTINE
- ATE HEALTHY WHOLE FOODS
- READ AT LEAST 10 PAGES OF ANY BOOK

REFLECTIION:

_____
_____
_____
_____
_____
_____
_____
_____
_____

TODAY'S AFFIRMATION

GRATITUDE
SHIFTS MY ENERGY
AND
BRINGS ME MORE
OF
WHAT I DESIRE

The Art of Becoming

DAY 139

DAILY CHECK IN: ✓

- WOKE UP EARLY
- WENT TO THE GYM
- MORNING ROUTINE
- NIGHT ROUTINE
- ATE HEALTHY WHOLE FOODS
- READ AT LEAST 10 PAGES OF ANY BOOK

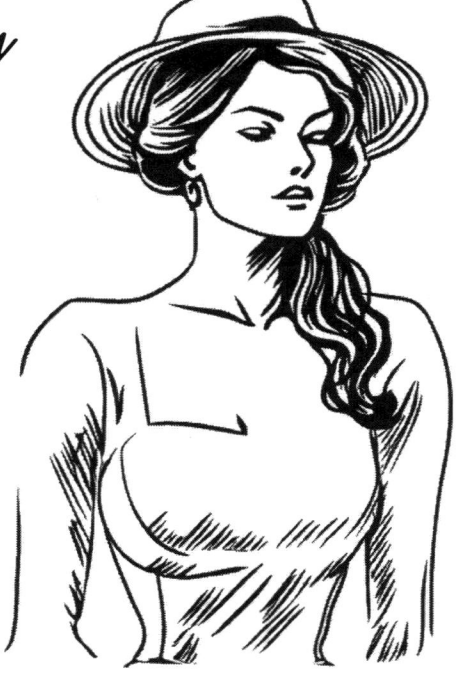

REFLECTIION:

_____
_____
_____
_____
_____
_____
_____
_____
_____

TODAY'S AFFIRMATION

EVERY VERSION OF ME HAS SERVED A PURPOSE IN MY EVOLUTION

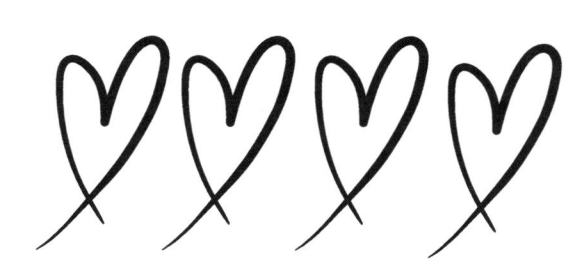

DAY 140

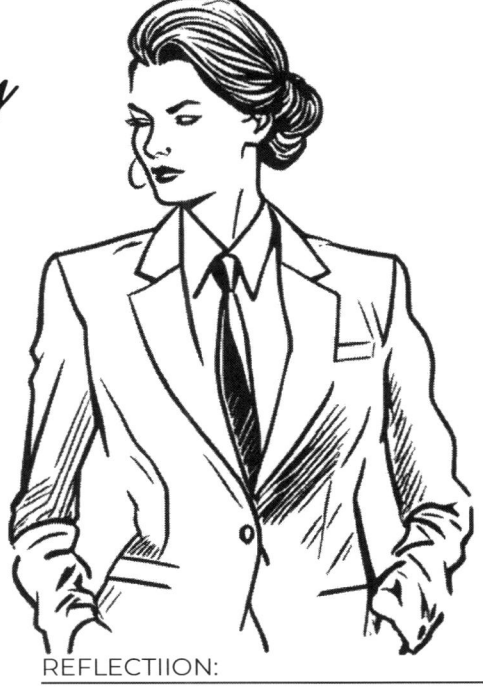

The Art of Becoming

DAILY CHECK IN: ✓

- WOKE UP EARLY
- WENT TO THE GYM
- MORNING ROUTINE
- NIGHT ROUTINE
- ATE HEALTHY WHOLE FOODS
- READ AT LEAST 10 PAGES OF ANY BOOK

REFLECTIION:

_____
_____
_____
_____
_____
_____
_____
_____
_____

TODAY'S AFFIRMATION

I CHOOSE TO LIVE EACH DAY WITH PURPOSE AND PASSION

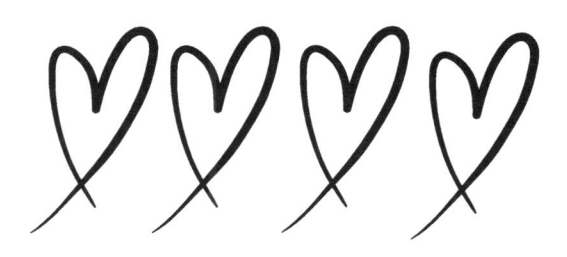

DAY 141

The Art of Becoming

DAILY CHECK IN: ✓

- WOKE UP EARLY
- WENT TO THE GYM
- MORNING ROUTINE
- NIGHT ROUTINE
- ATE HEALTHY WHOLE FOODS
- READ AT LEAST 10 PAGES OF ANY BOOK

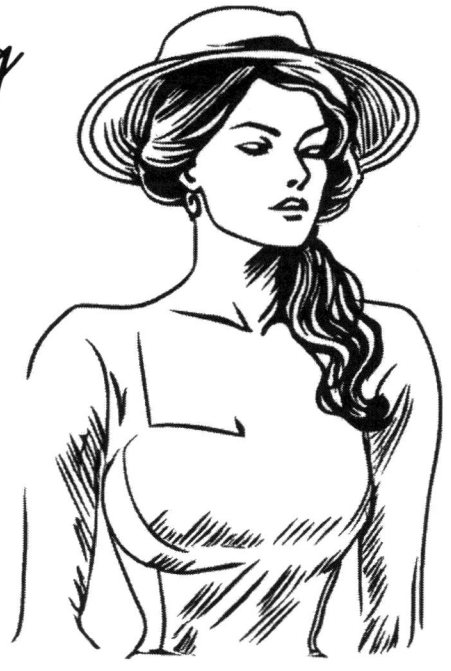

REFLECTIION:

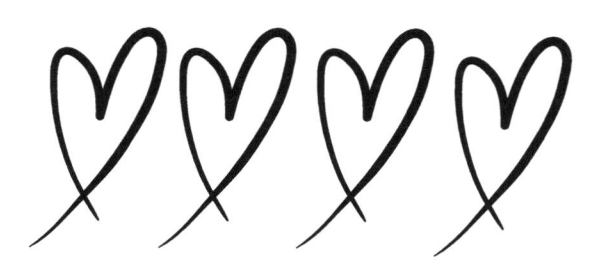

_____
_____
_____
_____
_____
_____
_____
_____
_____

TODAY'S AFFIRMATION

I DESERVE THE BEST, AND I WELCOME IT INTO MY LIFE

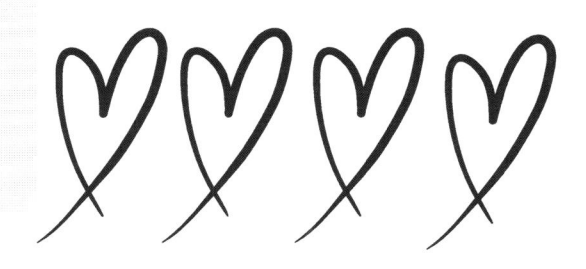

The Art of Becoming

DAY 142

DAILY CHECK IN: ✓

- WOKE UP EARLY ☐
- WENT TO THE GYM ☐
- MORNING ROUTINE ☐
- NIGHT ROUTINE ☐
- ATE HEALTHY WHOLE FOODS ☐
- READ AT LEAST 10 PAGES OF ANY BOOK ☐

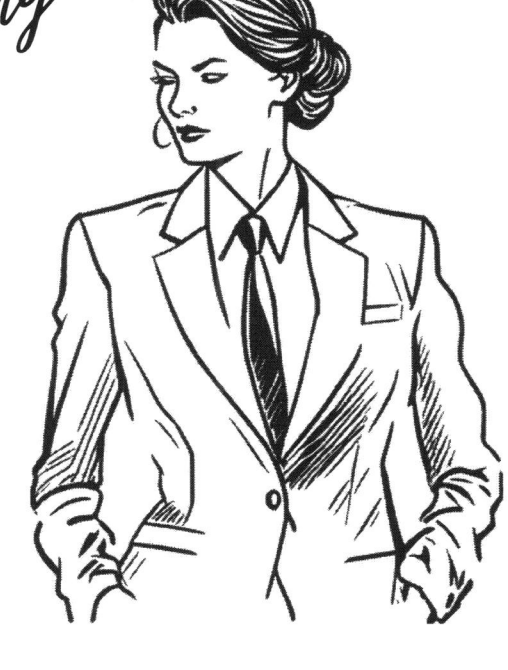

REFLECTIION:

_____
_____
_____
_____
_____
_____
_____
_____
_____

TODAY'S AFFIRMATION

I TAKE CARE OF MYSELF EMOTIONALLY, PHYSICALLY, AND SPIRITUALLY

♥ ♥ ♥ ♥

The Art of Becoming

DAY 143

DAILY CHECK IN: ✓

- WOKE UP EARLY
- WENT TO THE GYM
- MORNING ROUTINE
- NIGHT ROUTINE
- ATE HEALTHY WHOLE FOODS
- READ AT LEAST 10 PAGES OF ANY BOOK

REFLECTIION:

_____
_____
_____
_____
_____
_____
_____
_____
_____

TODAY'S AFFIRMATION

I ATTRACT POSITIVE, HIGH-VALUE RELATIONSHIPS

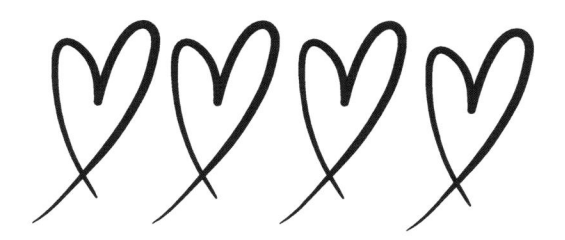

The Art of Becoming

DAY 144

DAILY CHECK IN: ✓

- WOKE UP EARLY
- WENT TO THE GYM
- MORNING ROUTINE
- NIGHT ROUTINE
- ATE HEALTHY WHOLE FOODS
- READ AT LEAST 10 PAGES OF ANY BOOK

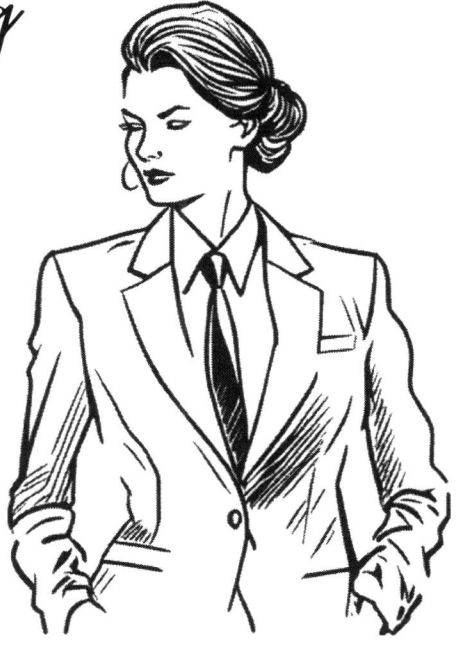

REFLECTIION:

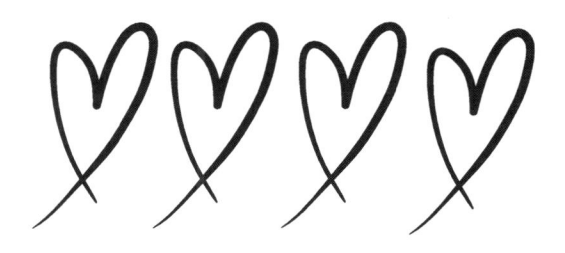

_____
_____
_____
_____
_____
_____
_____
_____

TODAY'S AFFIRMATION

I AM DEEPLY LOVED AND CHERISHED BY THOSE AROUND ME

The Art of Becoming

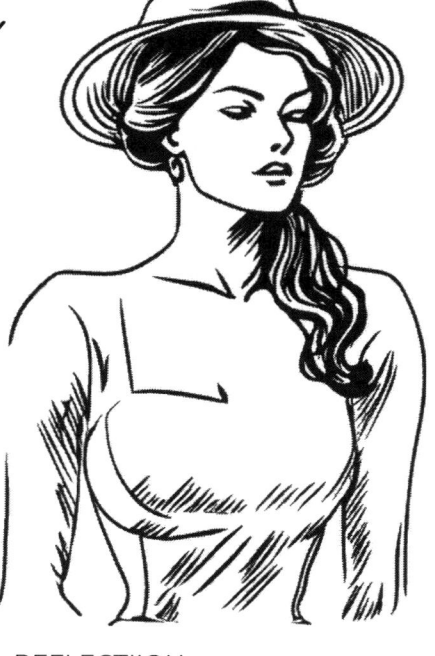

DAY 145

DAILY CHECK IN: ✓

- WOKE UP EARLY
- WENT TO THE GYM
- MORNING ROUTINE
- NIGHT ROUTINE
- ATE HEALTHY WHOLE FOODS
- READ AT LEAST 10 PAGES OF ANY BOOK

REFLECTIION:

_____
_____
_____
_____
_____
_____
_____
_____
_____
_____

TODAY'S AFFIRMATION

I AM ENOUGH, JUST AS I AM

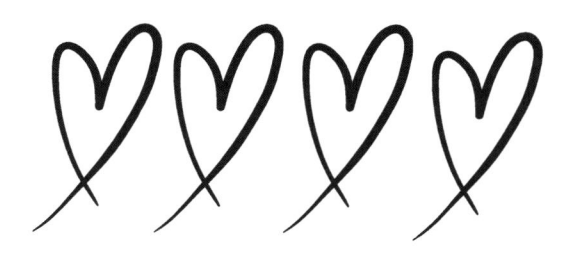

DAY 146

The Art of Becoming

DAILY CHECK IN: ✓

- WOKE UP EARLY
- WENT TO THE GYM
- MORNING ROUTINE
- NIGHT ROUTINE
- ATE HEALTHY WHOLE FOODS
- READ AT LEAST 10 PAGES OF ANY BOOK

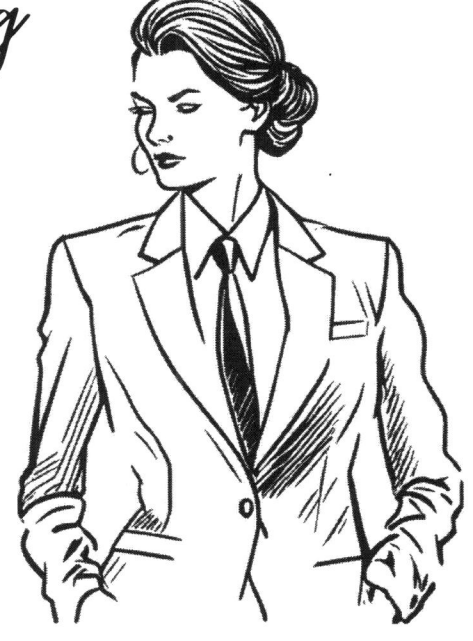

REFLECTIION:

_____
_____
_____
_____
_____
_____
_____
_____
_____

TODAY'S AFFIRMATION

I EMBRACE MY NATURAL BEAUTY AND RADIANCE

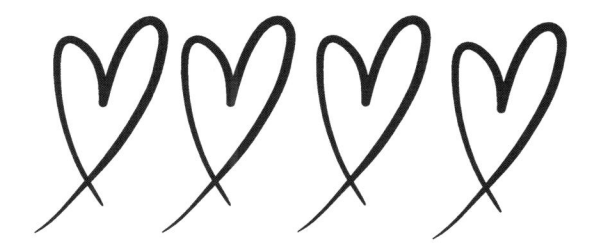

The Art of Becoming

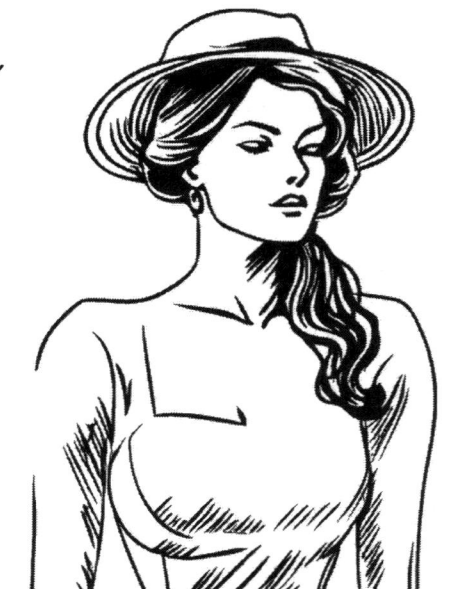

DAY 147

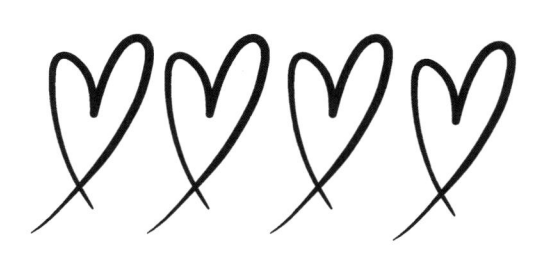

DAILY CHECK IN: ✓

- WOKE UP EARLY ☐
- WENT TO THE GYM ☐
- MORNING ROUTINE ☐
- NIGHT ROUTINE ☐
- ATE HEALTHY WHOLE FOODS ☐
- READ AT LEAST 10 PAGES OF ANY BOOK ☐

TODAY'S AFFIRMATION

I TAKE FULL RESPONSIBILTY FOR MY OWN HAPPINESS

REFLECTIION:

_____
_____
_____
_____
_____
_____
_____
_____
_____

The Art of Becoming

DAY 148

DAILY CHECK IN: ✓

- WOKE UP EARLY
- WENT TO THE GYM
- MORNING ROUTINE
- NIGHT ROUTINE
- ATE HEALTHY WHOLE FOODS
- READ AT LEAST 10 PAGES OF ANY BOOK

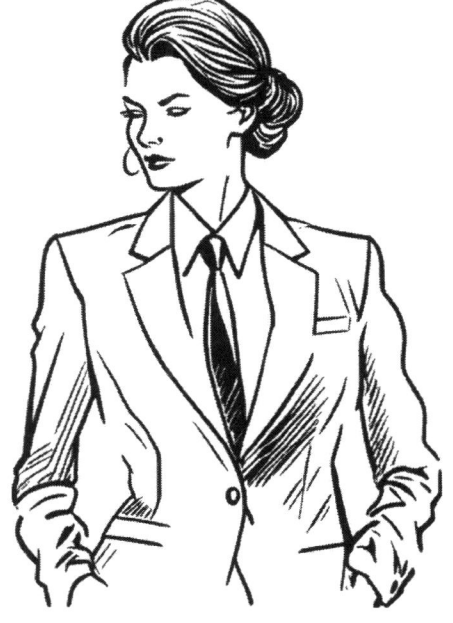

REFLECTIION:

_____
_____
_____
_____
_____
_____
_____
_____
_____

TODAY'S AFFIRMATION

I
AM
AM INPIRATION
TO
OTHERS

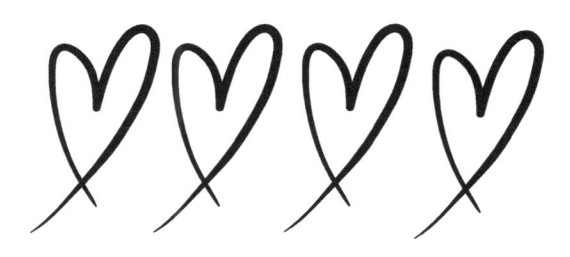

The Art of Becoming

DAY 149

DAILY CHECK IN: ✓

- WOKE UP EARLY
- WENT TO THE GYM
- MORNING ROUTINE
- NIGHT ROUTINE
- ATE HEALTHY WHOLE FOODS
- READ AT LEAST 10 PAGES OF ANY BOOK

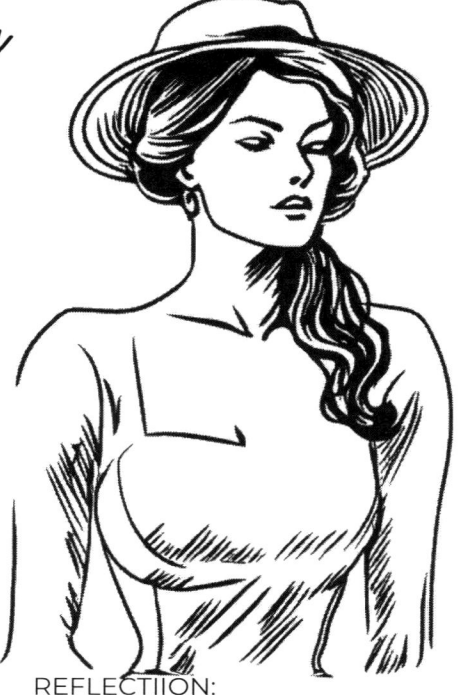

REFLECTIION:

_____
_____
_____
_____
_____
_____
_____
_____
_____

TODAY'S AFFIRMATION

I TRUST MY INTUITION AND ALLOW IT TO GUIDE ME

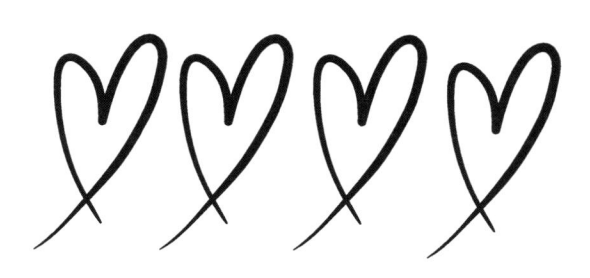

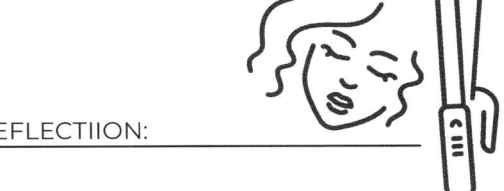

The Art of Becoming

DAY 150

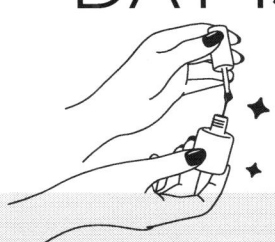

MAINTENANCE DAY
TIME
TO VISIT
THE
BEAUTY PARLOR
BABES!

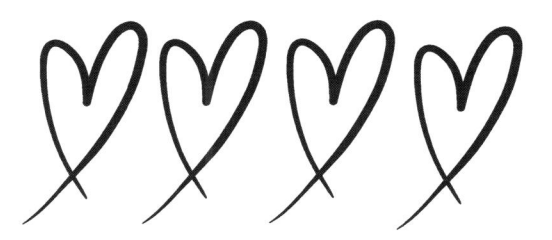

DAILY CHECK IN: ✓

- WOKE UP EARLY
- WENT TO THE GYM
- MORNING ROUTINE
- NIGHT ROUTINE
- ATE HEALTHY WHOLE FOODS
- READ AT LEAST 10 PAGES OF ANY BOOK

REFLECTIION:

_____
_____
_____
_____
_____
_____
_____
_____
_____

TODAY'S AFFIRMATION

I
LOVE
THE WOMAN
I AM
BECOMING

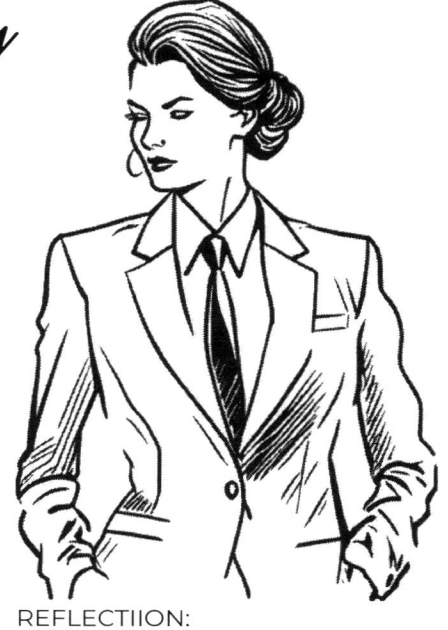

The Art of Becoming

DAY 151

DAILY CHECK IN: ✓

- WOKE UP EARLY
- WENT TO THE GYM
- MORNING ROUTINE
- NIGHT ROUTINE
- ATE HEALTHY WHOLE FOODS
- READ AT LEAST 10 PAGES OF ANY BOOK

REFLECTIION:
_____
_____
_____
_____
_____
_____
_____
_____
_____

TODAY'S AFFIRMATION

I
ALLOW MYSELF
TO
SHINE
UNAPOLOGETICALLY

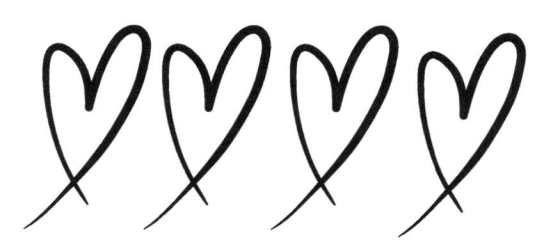

DAY 152

The Art of Becoming

DAILY CHECK IN: ✓

- WOKE UP EARLY
- WENT TO THE GYM
- MORNING ROUTINE
- NIGHT ROUTINE
- ATE HEALTHY WHOLE FOODS
- READ AT LEAST 10 PAGES OF ANY BOOK

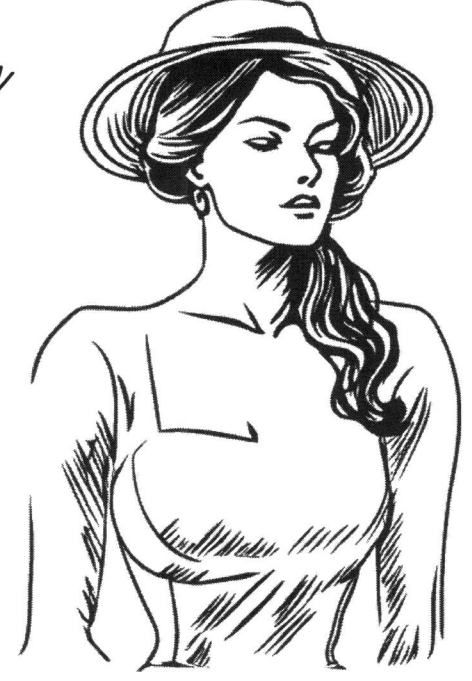

REFLECTIION:

_____
_____
_____
_____
_____
_____
_____
_____

TODAY'S AFFIRMATION

I
AM
THE CREATOR
OF MY OWN
HAPPINESS

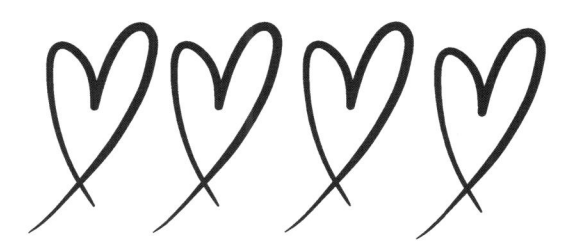

The Art of Becoming

DAY 153

DAILY CHECK IN: ✓

- WOKE UP EARLY ☐
- WENT TO THE GYM ☐
- MORNING ROUTINE ☐
- NIGHT ROUTINE ☐
- ATE HEALTHY WHOLE FOODS ☐
- READ AT LEAST 10 PAGES OF ANY BOOK ☐

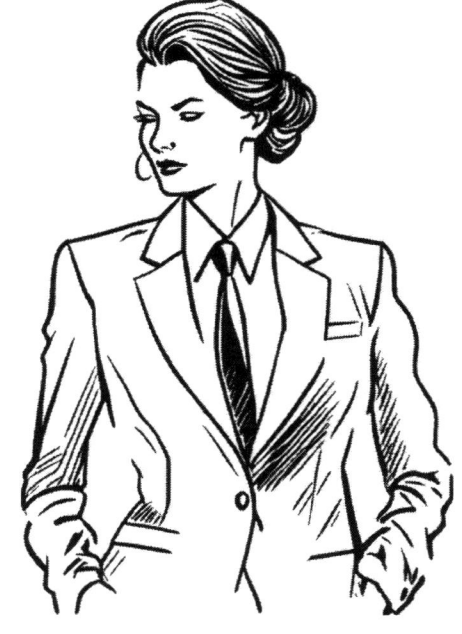

REFLECTIION:

_____
_____
_____
_____
_____
_____
_____
_____
_____

TODAY'S AFFIRMATION

I TRUST IN MY OWN CAPABILITIES

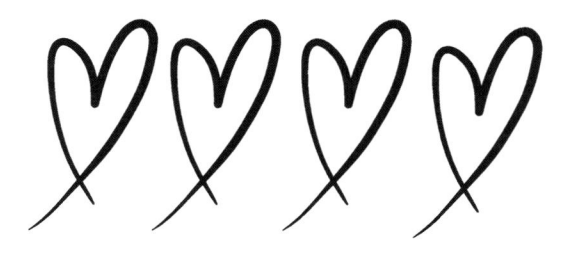

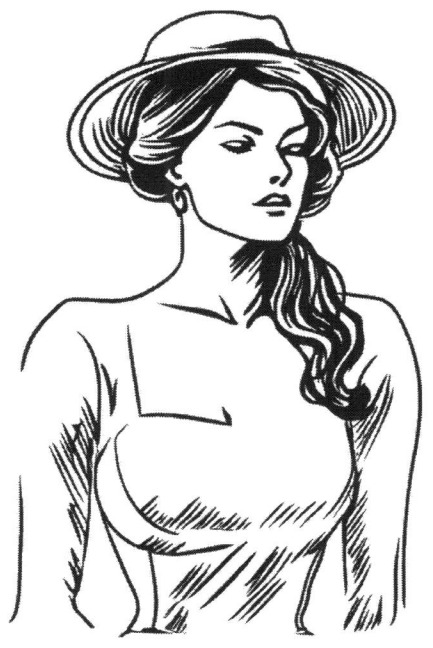

The Art of Becoming

DAY 154

DAILY CHECK IN: ✓

- WOKE UP EARLY
- WENT TO THE GYM
- MORNING ROUTINE
- NIGHT ROUTINE
- ATE HEALTHY WHOLE FOODS
- READ AT LEAST 10 PAGES OF ANY BOOK

REFLECTIION:

_____
_____
_____
_____
_____
_____
_____
_____
_____

TODAY'S AFFIRMATION

I
AM A WOMAN
OF
HIGH VALUE
AND
HIGH STANDARDS

DAY 155

The Art of Becoming

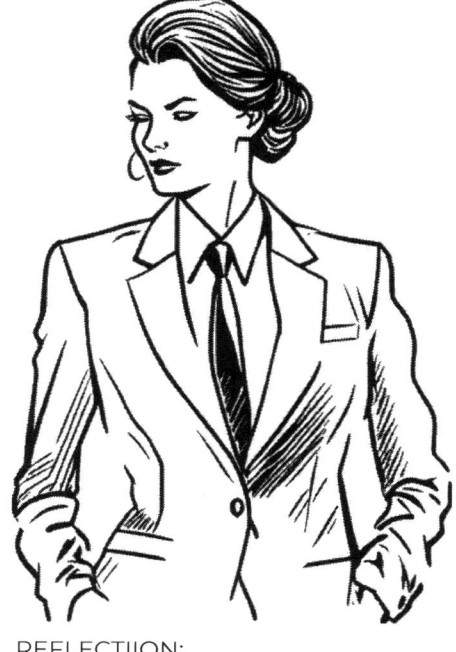

DAILY CHECK IN: ✓

- WOKE UP EARLY
- WENT TO THE GYM
- MORNING ROUTINE
- NIGHT ROUTINE
- ATE HEALTHY WHOLE FOODS
- READ AT LEAST 10 PAGES OF ANY BOOK

REFLECTIION:

_____
_____
_____
_____
_____
_____
_____
_____
_____
_____

TODAY'S AFFIRMATION

I EMBRACE MY WORTHINESS IN EVERY ASPECT OF LIFE

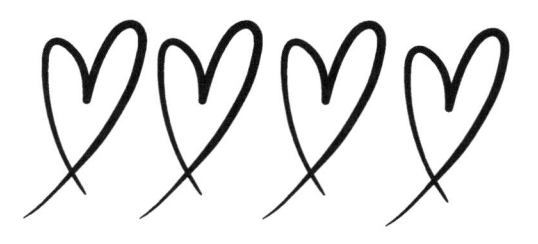

The Art of Becoming

DAY 156

DAILY CHECK IN: ✓

- WOKE UP EARLY
- WENT TO THE GYM
- MORNING ROUTINE
- NIGHT ROUTINE
- ATE HEALTHY WHOLE FOODS
- READ AT LEAST 10 PAGES OF ANY BOOK

REFLECTIION:

_____
_____
_____
_____
_____
_____
_____
_____

TODAY'S AFFIRMATION

I AM EXACTLY WHERE I NEED TO BE

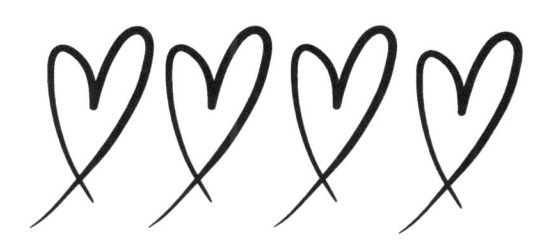

DAY 157

The Art of Becoming

__DAILY CHECK IN:__ ✓

- WOKE UP EARLY
- WENT TO THE GYM
- MORNING ROUTINE
- NIGHT ROUTINE
- ATE HEALTHY WHOLE FOODS
- READ AT LEAST 10 PAGES OF ANY BOOK

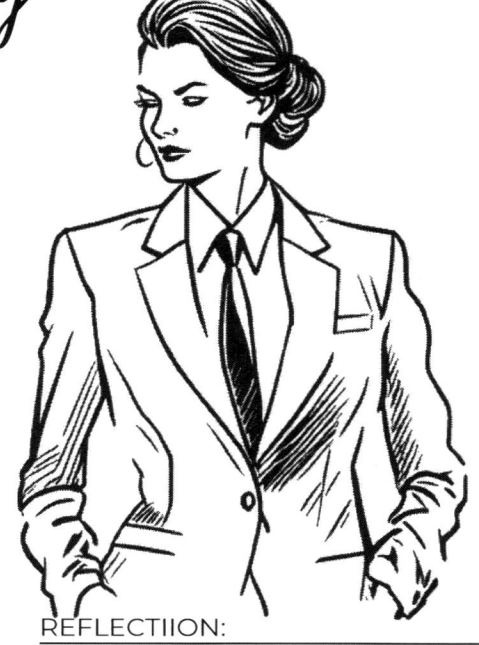

__REFLECTIION:__

_____
_____
_____
_____
_____
_____
_____
_____
_____

__TODAY'S AFFIRMATION__

I MOVE FOWARD WITH FAITH, CONFIDENCE, AND EXCITEMENT

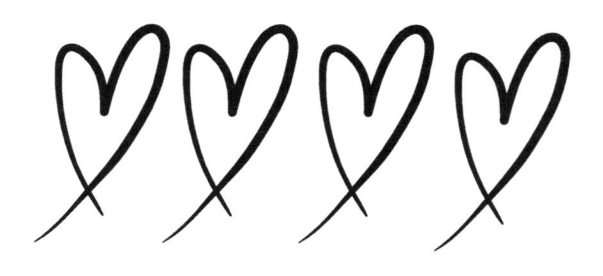

The Art of Becoming

DAY 158

DAILY CHECK IN: ✓

- WOKE UP EARLY
- WENT TO THE GYM
- MORNING ROUTINE
- NIGHT ROUTINE
- ATE HEALTHY WHOLE FOODS
- READ AT LEAST 10 PAGES OF ANY BOOK

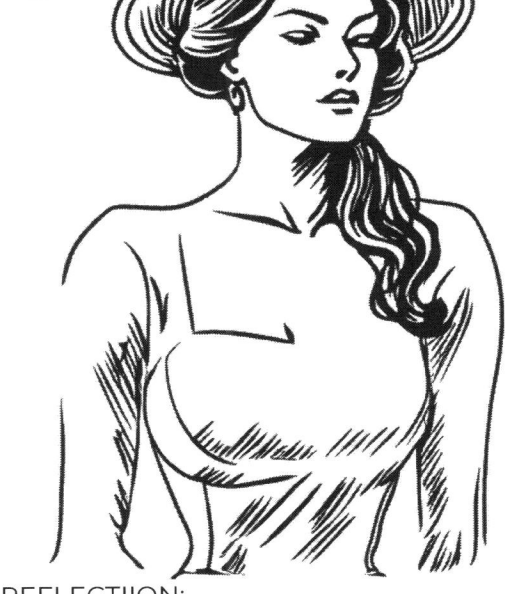

REFLECTIION:

___

TODAY'S AFFIRMATION

I AM UNSTOPPABLE, FEARLESS, AND LIMITLESS

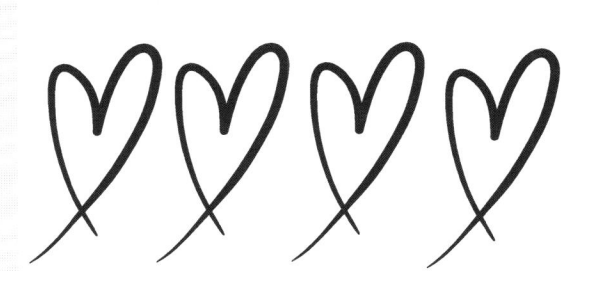

The Art of Becoming

DAY 159

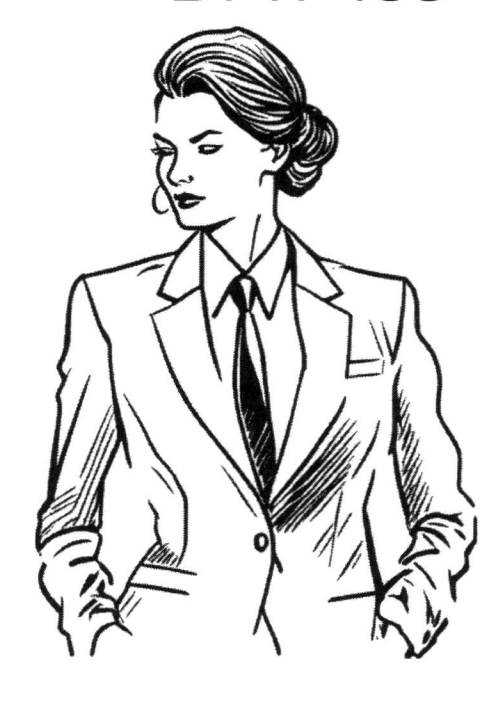

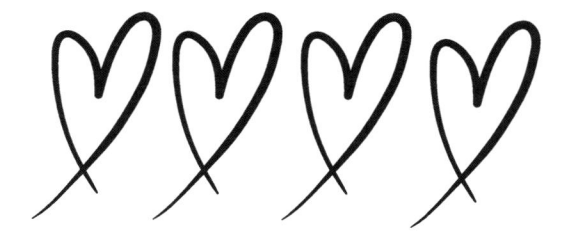

DAILY CHECK IN: ✓

- WOKE UP EARLY ☐
- WENT TO THE GYM ☐
- MORNING ROUTINE ☐
- NIGHT ROUTINE ☐
- ATE HEALTHY WHOLE FOODS ☐
- READ AT LEAST 10 PAGES OF ANY BOOK ☐

REFLECTIION:
_____
_____
_____
_____
_____
_____
_____
_____
_____

TODAY'S AFFIRMATION

I AM CAPABLE OF GROWTH AND CHANGE

♡ ♡ ♡ ♡

The Art of Becoming

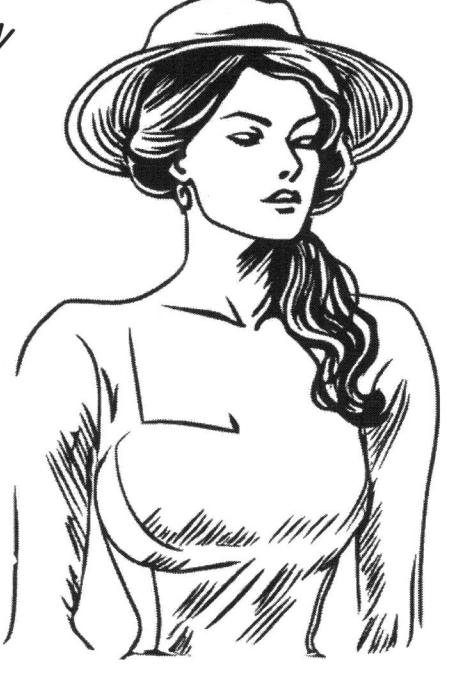

DAY 160

DAILY CHECK IN: ✓

- WOKE UP EARLY
- WENT TO THE GYM
- MORNING ROUTINE
- NIGHT ROUTINE
- ATE HEALTHY WHOLE FOODS
- READ AT LEAST 10 PAGES OF ANY BOOK

REFLECTIION:
_____
_____
_____
_____
_____
_____
_____
_____
_____

TODAY'S AFFIRMATION

I TRUST MYSELF TO MAKE WISE DECISIONS

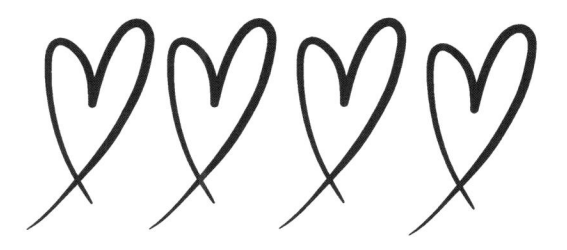

The Art of Becoming

DAY 161

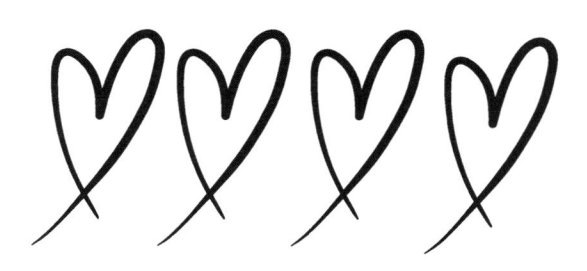

DAILY CHECK IN: ✓

- WOKE UP EARLY
- WENT TO THE GYM
- MORNING ROUTINE
- NIGHT ROUTINE
- ATE HEALTHY WHOLE FOODS
- READ AT LEAST 10 PAGES OF ANY BOOK

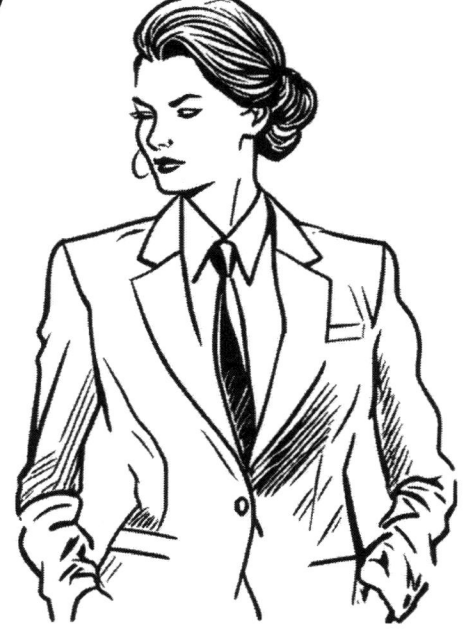

REFLECTIION:

_____
_____
_____
_____
_____
_____
_____
_____
_____
_____

TODAY'S AFFIRMATION

I
AM
STRONG
AND
RESILIENT

The Art of Becoming

DAY 162

DAILY CHECK IN: ✓

- WOKE UP EARLY
- WENT TO THE GYM
- MORNING ROUTINE
- NIGHT ROUTINE
- ATE HEALTHY WHOLE FOODS
- READ AT LEAST 10 PAGES OF ANY BOOK

REFLECTIION:

_____
_____
_____
_____
_____
_____
_____
_____

TODAY'S AFFIRMATION

I CELEBRATE MY UNIQUE STRENGHTS AND TALENTS

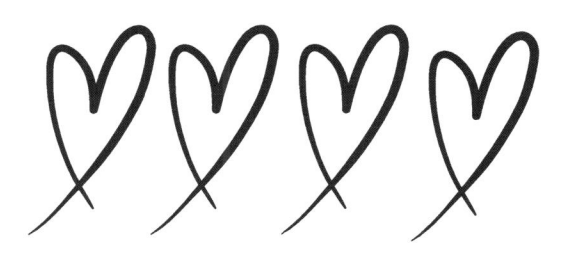

The Art of Becoming

DAY 163

DAILY CHECK IN: ✓

- WOKE UP EARLY ☐
- WENT TO THE GYM ☐
- MORNING ROUTINE ☐
- NIGHT ROUTINE ☐
- ATE HEALTHY WHOLE FOODS ☐
- READ AT LEAST 10 PAGES OF ANY BOOK ☐

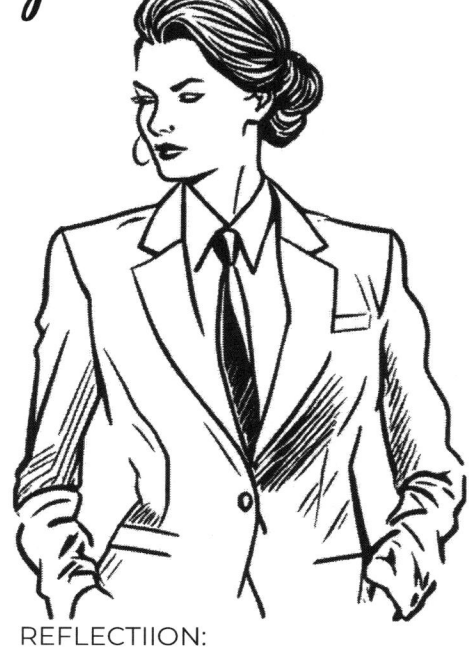

REFLECTIION:

_____
_____
_____
_____
_____
_____
_____
_____
_____

TODAY'S AFFIRMATION

I AM WORTHY OF LOVE, CARE, AND RESPECT - FROM MYSELF AND OTHERS

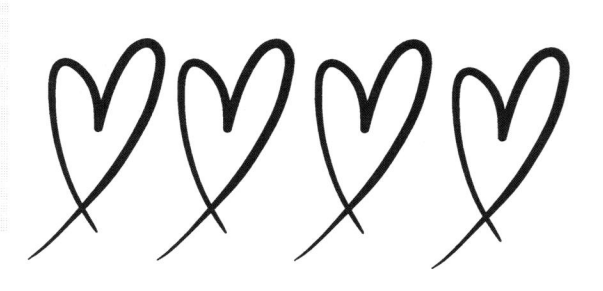

The Art of Becoming

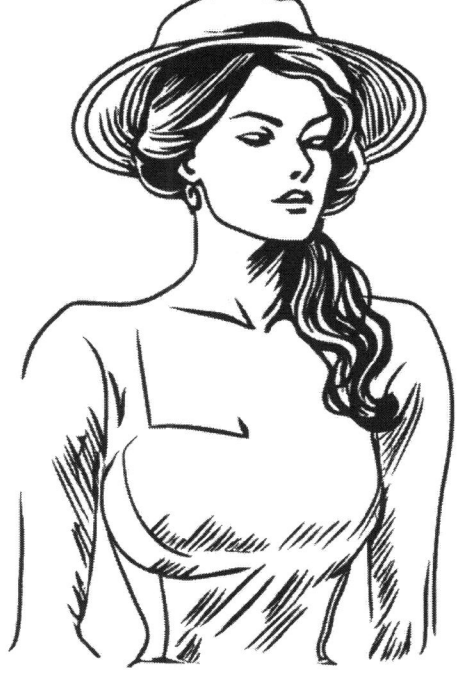

DAY 164

DAILY CHECK IN: ✓

- WOKE UP EARLY
- WENT TO THE GYM
- MORNING ROUTINE
- NIGHT ROUTINE
- ATE HEALTHY WHOLE FOODS
- READ AT LEAST 10 PAGES OF ANY BOOK

REFLECTIION:

_____
_____
_____
_____
_____
_____
_____
_____
_____

TODAY'S AFFIRMATION

I COMMIT TO LEARNING AND SELF-IMPROVEMENT EVERY DAY

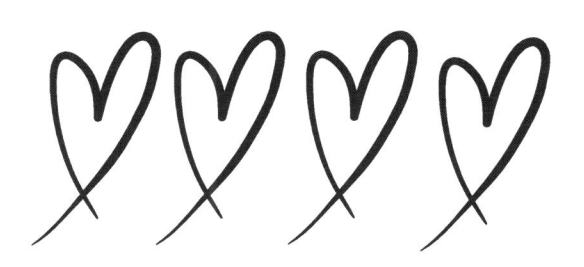

DAY 165

The Art of Becoming

DAILY CHECK IN: ✓

- WOKE UP EARLY ☐
- WENT TO THE GYM ☐
- MORNING ROUTINE ☐
- NIGHT ROUTINE ☐
- ATE HEALTHY WHOLE FOODS ☐
- READ AT LEAST 10 PAGES OF ANY BOOK ☐

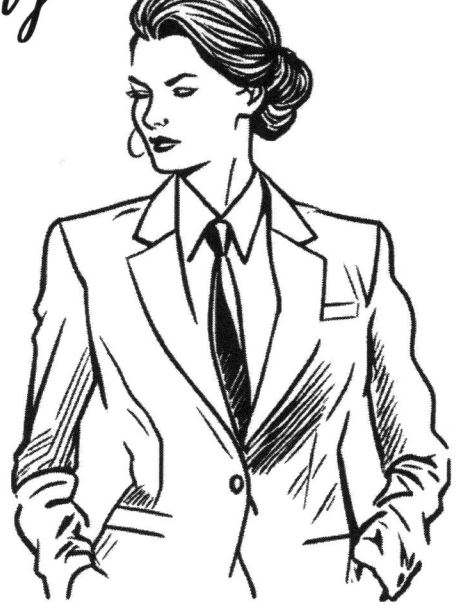

REFLECTIION:

_____
_____
_____
_____
_____
_____
_____
_____

TODAY'S AFFIRMATION

I AM PATIENT AND KIND TO MYSELF AS I GROW

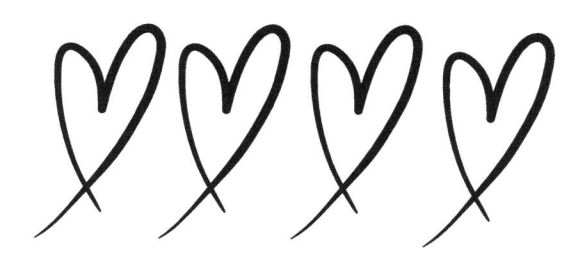

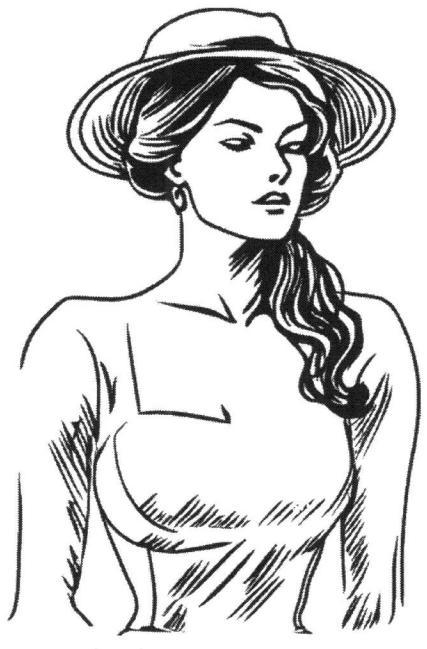

The Art of Becoming

DAY 166

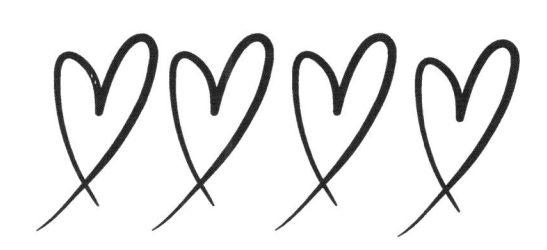

DAILY CHECK IN: ✓

- WOKE UP EARLY
- WENT TO THE GYM
- MORNING ROUTINE
- NIGHT ROUTINE
- ATE HEALTHY WHOLE FOODS
- READ AT LEAST 10 PAGES OF ANY BOOK

REFLECTIION:

_____
_____
_____
_____
_____
_____
_____
_____
_____

TODAY'S AFFIRMATION

I FOCUS ON PROGRESS, NOT PERFECTION

The Art of Becoming

DAY 167

DAILY CHECK IN: ✓

- WOKE UP EARLY ☐
- WENT TO THE GYM ☐
- MORNING ROUTINE ☐
- NIGHT ROUTINE ☐
- ATE HEALTHY WHOLE FOODS ☐
- READ AT LEAST 10 PAGES OF ANY BOOK ☐

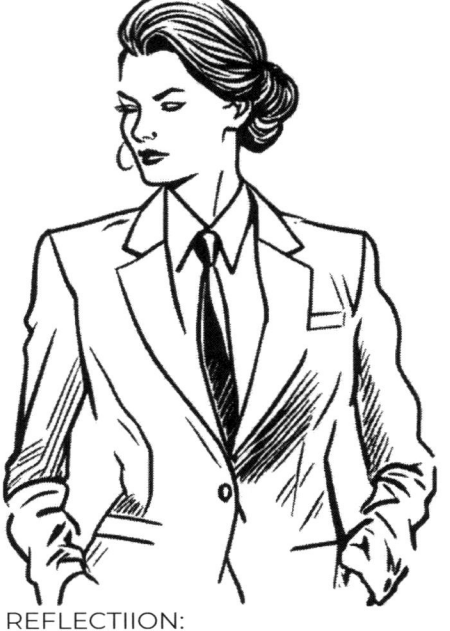

REFLECTIION: _____
_____
_____
_____
_____
_____
_____
_____
_____

TODAY'S AFFIRMATION

I AM GRATEFUL FOR THE OPPORTUNITIES TO LEARN AND GROW

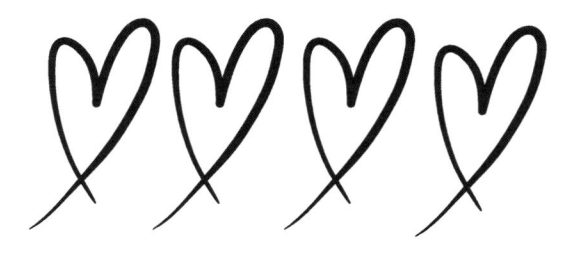

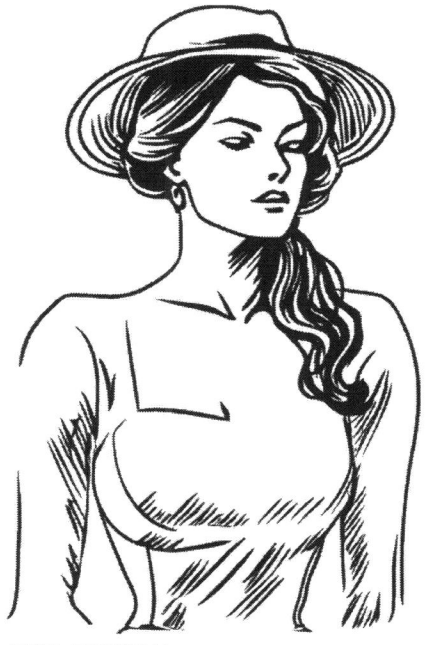

The Art of Becoming

DAY 168

DAILY CHECK IN: ✓

- WOKE UP EARLY ☐
- WENT TO THE GYM ☐
- MORNING ROUTINE ☐
- NIGHT ROUTINE ☐
- ATE HEALTHY WHOLE FOODS ☐
- READ AT LEAST 10 PAGES OF ANY BOOK ☐

REFLECTIION: _____
_____
_____
_____
_____
_____
_____
_____
_____

TODAY'S AFFIRMATION

I TAKE OWNERSHIP OF MY MISTAKES AND USE THEM AS LESSONS

♡ ♡ ♡ ♡

DAY 169

The Art of Becoming

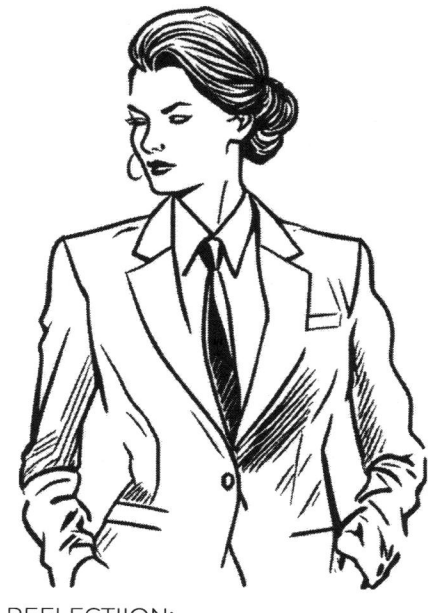

DAILY CHECK IN: ✓

- WOKE UP EARLY
- WENT TO THE GYM
- MORNING ROUTINE
- NIGHT ROUTINE
- ATE HEALTHY WHOLE FOODS
- READ AT LEAST 10 PAGES OF ANY BOOK

REFLECTIION:

_____
_____
_____
_____
_____
_____
_____
_____
_____
_____

TODAY'S AFFIRMATION

I CHOOSE TO FOCUS ON THE POSITIVE ASPECTS OF MY LIFE

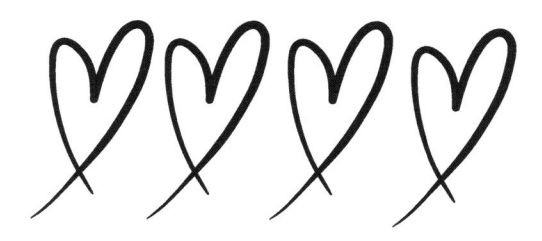

The Art of Becoming

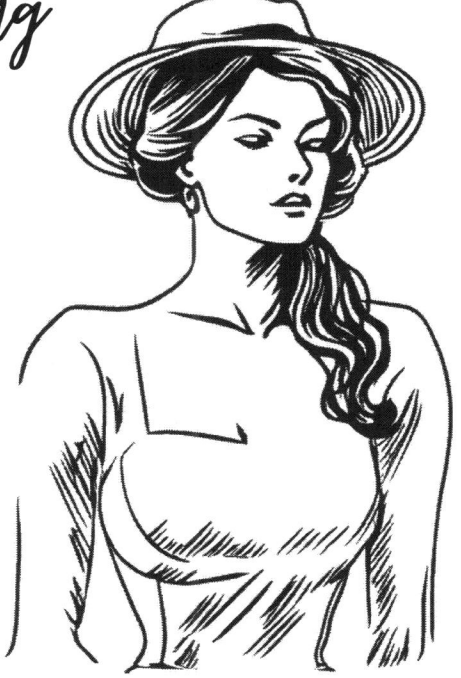

DAY 170

DAILY CHECK IN: ✓

- WOKE UP EARLY
- WENT TO THE GYM
- MORNING ROUTINE
- NIGHT ROUTINE
- ATE HEALTHY WHOLE FOODS
- READ AT LEAST 10 PAGES OF ANY BOOK

REFLECTIION:
_____
_____
_____
_____
_____
_____
_____
_____
_____

TODAY'S AFFIRMATION

I
AM MOTIVATED
TO
ACHIEVE MY GOALS
AND
DREAMS

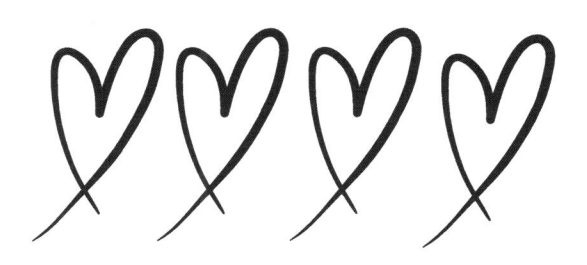

DAY 171

The Art of Becoming

DAILY CHECK IN: ✓

- WOKE UP EARLY
- WENT TO THE GYM
- MORNING ROUTINE
- NIGHT ROUTINE
- ATE HEALTHY WHOLE FOODS
- READ AT LEAST 10 PAGES OF ANY BOOK

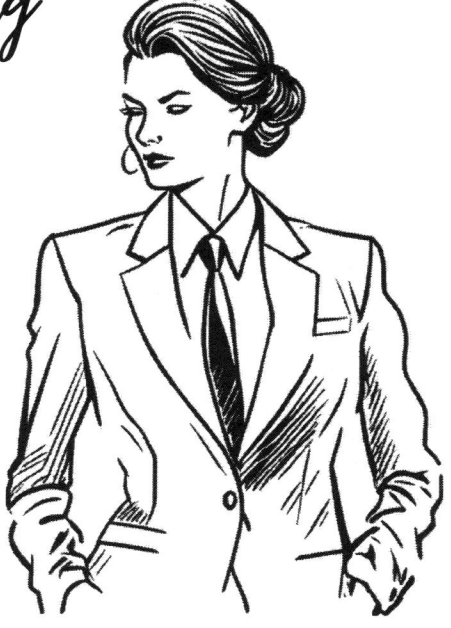

REFLECTIION:

_____
_____
_____
_____
_____
_____
_____
_____
_____

TODAY'S AFFIRMATION

I
BELIEVE
IN MY ABILTY
TO
SUCCEED

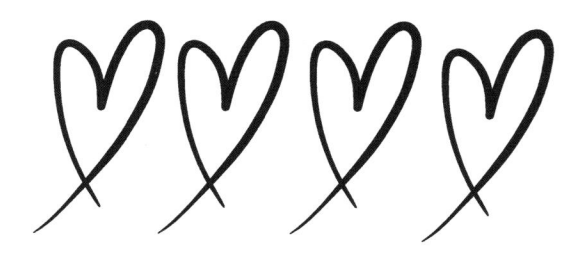

The Art of Becoming

DAY 172

DAILY CHECK IN: ✓

- WOKE UP EARLY
- WENT TO THE GYM
- MORNING ROUTINE
- NIGHT ROUTINE
- ATE HEALTHY WHOLE FOODS
- READ AT LEAST 10 PAGES OF ANY BOOK

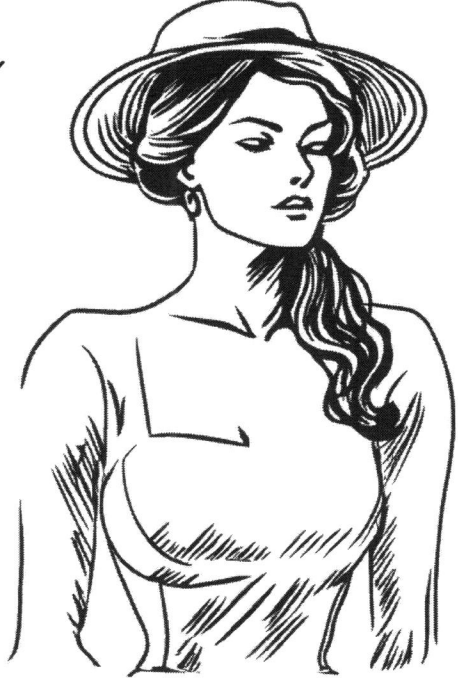

REFLECTIION:

_____
_____
_____
_____
_____
_____
_____
_____
_____

TODAY'S AFFIRMATION

I AM CONFIDENT IN MY SKILLS AND ABILITIES

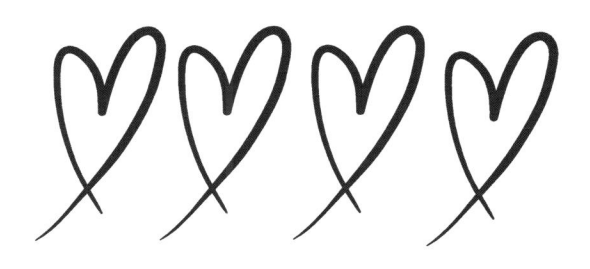

DAY 173

The Art of Becoming

DAILY CHECK IN: ✓

- WOKE UP EARLY
- WENT TO THE GYM
- MORNING ROUTINE
- NIGHT ROUTINE
- ATE HEALTHY WHOLE FOODS
- READ AT LEAST 10 PAGES OF ANY BOOK

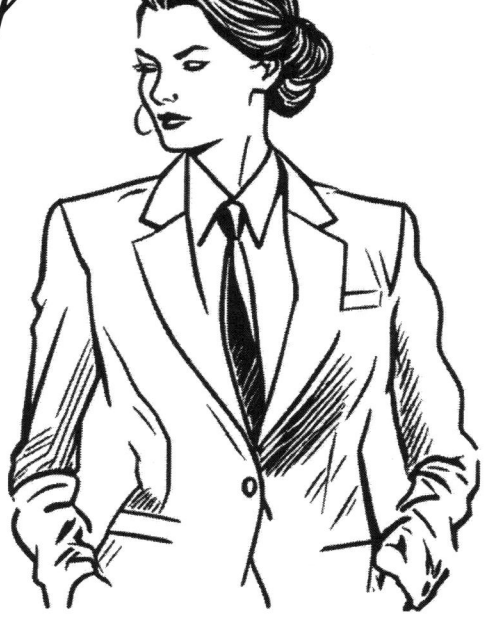

REFLECTIION:

_____
_____
_____
_____
_____
_____
_____
_____
_____

TODAY'S AFFIRMATION

I
TRUST
THAT EVERYTHING
WILL
WORK OUT
FOR MY
OWN GOOD

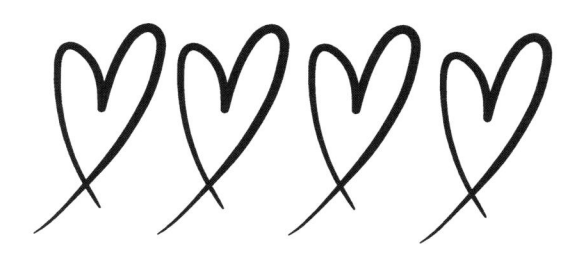

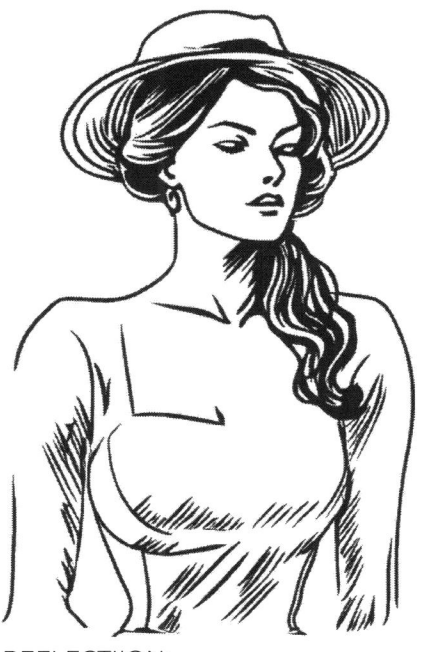

The Art of Becoming

DAY 174

DAILY CHECK IN: ✓

- WOKE UP EARLY
- WENT TO THE GYM
- MORNING ROUTINE
- NIGHT ROUTINE
- ATE HEALTHY WHOLE FOODS
- READ AT LEAST 10 PAGES OF ANY BOOK

REFLECTIION:

_____
_____
_____
_____
_____
_____
_____
_____
_____

TODAY'S AFFIRMATION

I ATTRACT POSITIVE, SUPPORTIVE RELATIONSHIPS INTO MY LIFE

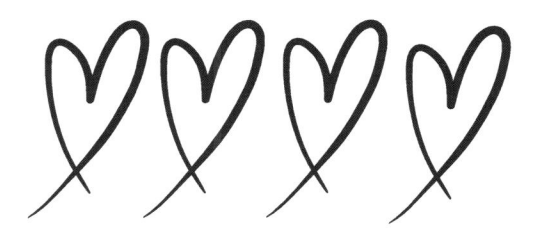

The Art of Becoming

DAY 175

DAILY CHECK IN: ✓

- WOKE UP EARLY ☐
- WENT TO THE GYM ☐
- MORNING ROUTINE ☐
- NIGHT ROUTINE ☐
- ATE HEALTHY WHOLE FOODS ☐
- READ AT LEAST 10 PAGES OF ANY BOOK ☐

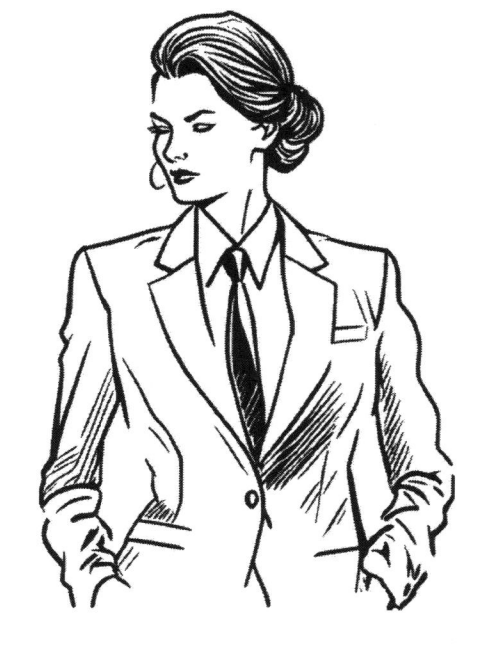

REFLECTIION:
_____
_____
_____
_____
_____
_____
_____
_____
_____
_____

TODAY'S AFFIRMATION

I AM GRATEFUL FOR THE LOVING PEOPLE IN MY LIFE

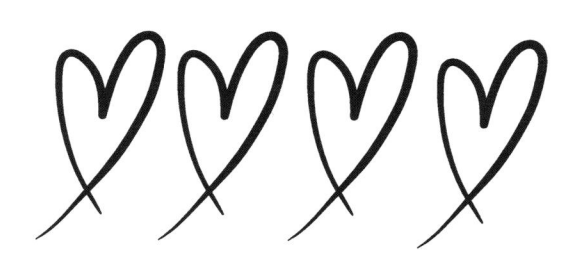

DAY 176

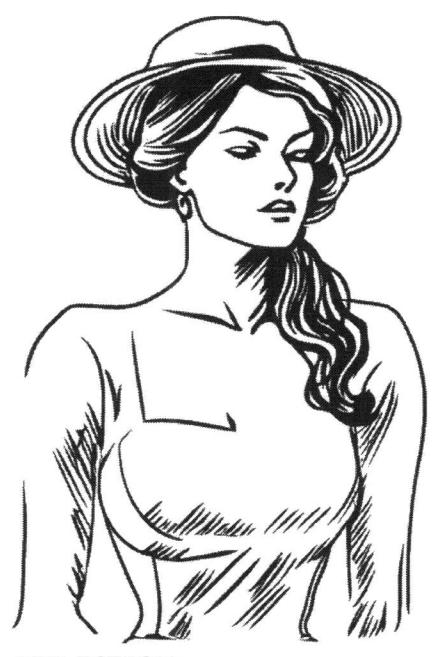

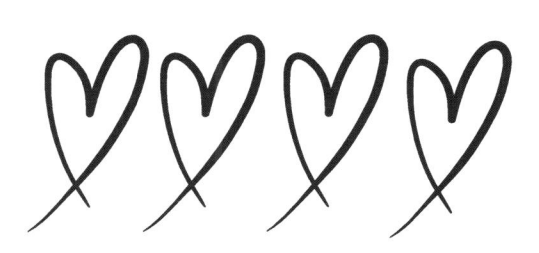

The Art of Becoming

DAILY CHECK IN: ✓

- WOKE UP EARLY
- WENT TO THE GYM
- MORNING ROUTINE
- NIGHT ROUTINE
- ATE HEALTHY WHOLE FOODS
- READ AT LEAST 10 PAGES OF ANY BOOK

REFLECTIION:

_____
_____
_____
_____
_____
_____
_____
_____
_____

TODAY'S AFFIRMATION

I COMMUNICATE EFFECTIVELY AND ASSERTIVELY

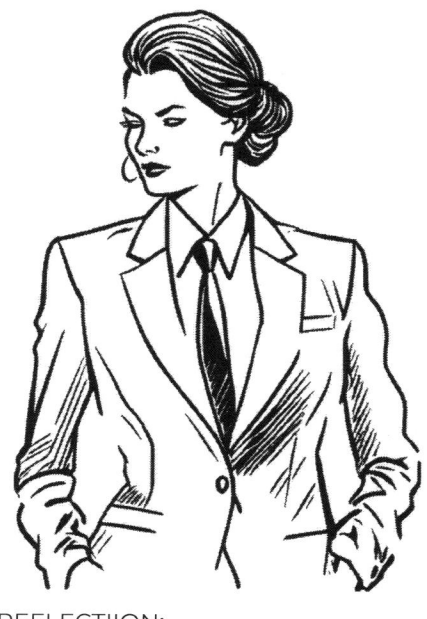

The Art of Becoming

DAY 177

DAILY CHECK IN: ✓

- WOKE UP EARLY ☐
- WENT TO THE GYM ☐
- MORNING ROUTINE ☐
- NIGHT ROUTINE ☐
- ATE HEALTHY WHOLE FOODS ☐
- READ AT LEAST 10 PAGES OF ANY BOOK ☐

REFLECTIION:
_____
_____
_____
_____
_____
_____
_____
_____
_____

TODAY'S AFFIRMATION

I NURTURE AND INVEST IN MY RELATIONSHIPS

The Art of Becoming

DAY 178

DAILY CHECK IN: ✓

- WOKE UP EARLY ☐
- WENT TO THE GYM ☐
- MORNING ROUTINE ☐
- NIGHT ROUTINE ☐
- ATE HEALTHY WHOLE FOODS ☐
- READ AT LEAST 10 PAGES OF ANY BOOK ☐

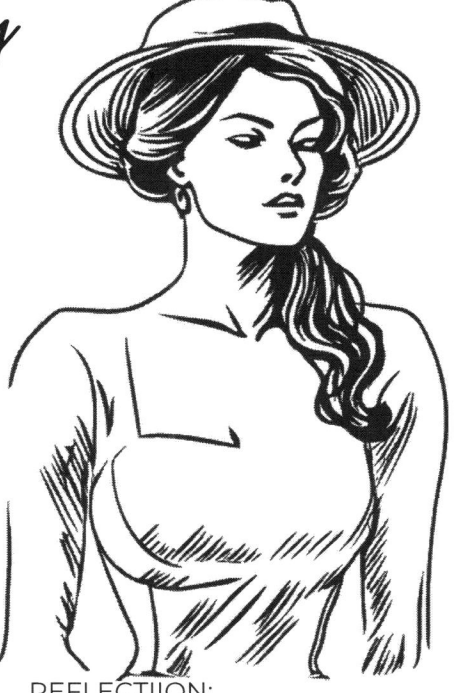

REFLECTIION:

_____
_____
_____
_____
_____
_____
_____
_____

TODAY'S AFFIRMATION

I AM PART OF A COMMUNITY THAT UPLIFTS AND INPIRES ME

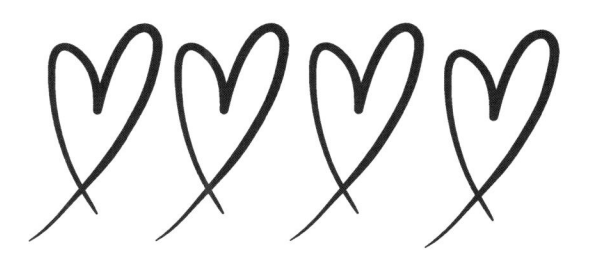

The Art of Becoming

DAY 179

DAILY CHECK IN: ✓

- WOKE UP EARLY
- WENT TO THE GYM
- MORNING ROUTINE
- NIGHT ROUTINE
- ATE HEALTHY WHOLE FOODS
- READ AT LEAST 10 PAGES OF ANY BOOK

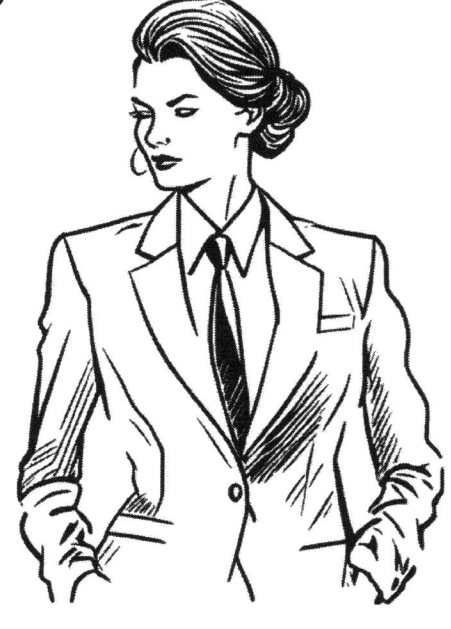

REFLECTIION:

_____
_____
_____
_____
_____
_____
_____
_____

TODAY'S AFFIRMATION

I RELEASE ALL LIMITATIONS AND DOUBTS, EMBRACING MY FULL POTENTIAL

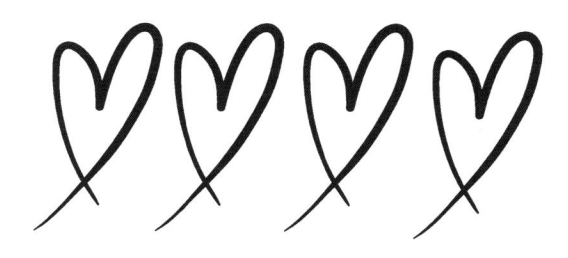

The Art of Becoming

DAY 180

DAILY CHECK IN: ✓

- WOKE UP EARLY
- WENT TO THE GYM
- MORNING ROUTINE
- NIGHT ROUTINE
- ATE HEALTHY WHOLE FOODS
- READ AT LEAST 10 PAGES OF ANY BOOK

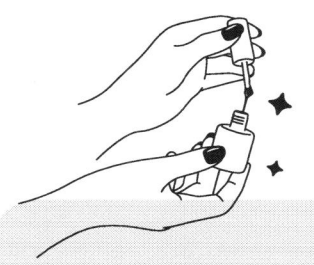

MAINTENANCE DAY
TIME
TO VISIT
THE BEAUTY PARLOR
,BABES!

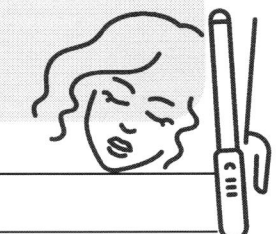

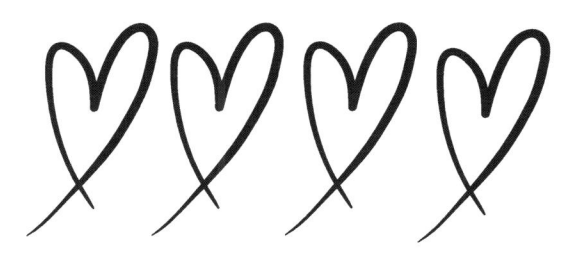

REFLECTIION:

_____

_____

_____

_____

_____

_____

_____

_____

TODAY'S AFFIRMATION

I
NOW KNOW
I AM
CAPABLE WITH
WHATEVER I SET
MY MIND ON

Made in the USA
Columbia, SC
15 April 2025

e4eabb39-57ad-4a33-8966-8b52ea0552d2R01